Vagus Nerve

Effective Self-Help Techniques and Stimulation Exercises to Activate Your Body's Healing Power. A Complete Guide to Break Free From Anxiety, Stress, Inflammation, Trauma and Sleep Disorder

© **Copyright 2019 - All rights reserved.**

The content contained within this book may not be reproduced, duplicated or transmitted without direct written permission from the author or the publisher.

Under no circumstances will any blame or legal responsibility be held against the publisher, or author, for any damages, reparation, or monetary loss due to the information contained within this book, either directly or indirectly.

Legal Notice:

This book is copyright protected. It is only for personal use. You cannot amend, distribute, sell, use, quote or paraphrase any part, or the content within this book, without the consent of the author or publisher.

Disclaimer Notice:

Please note the information contained within this document is for educational and entertainment purposes only. All effort has been executed to present accurate, up to date, reliable, complete information. No warranties of any kind are declared or implied. Readers acknowledge that the author is not engaging in the rendering of legal, financial, medical or professional advice. The content within this book has been derived from various sources. Please consult a licensed professional before attempting any techniques outlined in this book.

By reading this document, the reader agrees that under no circumstances is the author responsible for any losses, direct or indirect, that are incurred as a result of the use of the information contained within this document, including, but not limited to, errors, omissions, or inaccuracies.

Table of Contents

Chapter 1: The Vagus Nerve 8
   What Is the Vagus Nerve? 9
   What Does It Do? 10
      Effects on physiology 13
      Effects on mental health 17

Chapter 2: Fundamentals of Polyvagal Theory 23

Chapter 3: Vagus Nerve and Anxiety 27
   Social Anxiety 29
   Panic Disorder 31
   Generalized Anxiety Disorder 34
   Self-Help Strategies for Anxiety 38
      Immediate self-help strategies 39
      Long-term strategies 43

Chapter 4: Vagus Nerve and Trauma 51
   Self-Help Strategies for Trauma 63
      Immediate self-help strategies 65
      Long-term coping strategies 73

Chapter 5: Vagus Nerve and Depression 77
   Self-Help Strategies for Depression 81
      Cognitive distortions 81
      Relaxation techniques 88
      Exercise 95

Chapter 6: Stress, Inflammation, and Vagal Tone .100

Stress 101

Inflammation 102

Vagal Tone 104

Chapter 7: Techniques to Activate Your Vagus Nerve 107

Breathing Techniques 108

Mindfulness Meditation 113

Massage 121

Acupuncture 124

Change Your Diet 125

Supportive Relationships 126

Conclusion 128

References 129

Introduction

Imagine this. You're at work, sitting at your desk typing away. Next thing you know, you get a series of emails with notifications just popping up across your screen. Your boss is asking you why your work isn't done. Your boss needs this work now! With each frantic email, you start to feel stressed. You don't even have time to respond to the emails before another is received in the chain. The last email is the most ominous. Your boss would like to see you in their office.

For most people, experiencing a scenario like this will bring changes to your body. You'll feel like you're stressed. Your shoulders may be tense, you may start to sweat, and your heart rate may increase. With that last email, you may feel like your heart literally dropped to your stomach, with that peculiar swooping feeling. This is your body's normal reaction to stress, and it can be triggered by the most mundane life experiences, or the most traumatizing. Its constant activation leads to a whole host of mental health and physical issues.

Many adults in the U.S. struggle with their physical and mental well-being. It can be hard to work day by day with increasing stress levels while also accomplishing all of the things that we want in life. So how do we help ourselves succeed while also maintaining our mental and physical well-being? The answer is the vagus nerve.

Your vagus nerve can be the key to your well-being. It is a long nerve running through your body and touching most of your critical organs. It uses your environment to send signals from your brain to your organs and vice versa to determine whether or not you are safe and secure. In the situation above, if you know how to activate your vagus nerve, then you would know how to calm down so that when you do meet your boss, it's with a clear mind ready for decision-making. Activating your vagus nerve can protect you from a plethora of mental and physical issues in your life, from everyday stress to dealing with a traumatic stress response. Your vagus nerve can help you achieve wellness in your life.

This book will explore more about the vagus nerve and how it works throughout your body. It will discuss how it works in conjunction with your autonomic nervous system and how that, in turn, controls your body's reaction to your environment. From there it will discuss some various challenges to our mental and physical well-being. It will also discuss self-help techniques for specific difficulties to help us activate the vagus nerve and stay relaxed and calm. In essence, this book is your guide to the wandering nerve.

Chapter 1:
The Vagus Nerve

Imagine that your body is a country and you want to explore it starting from a major city and heading south. You stop to see all the sights and important cultural destinations. Sometimes you stick with one road and then turn back when the road ends. Then you choose another road to follow. When you travel like this, you often take branches off the main road, maybe explore some of the little side lanes, and maybe make a lot of U-turns! Eventually, you come to the end of the road, and the end of your wandering, but never the end of your adventure. This road map is similar to your nervous system.

Your nervous system has routes that start from your major "cities": your brain (cranial nerves) and your spinal cord (spinal nerves). Cranial nerves start from your brain and go in all sorts of directions, just like a road map from a big city. There are cranial nerves that only go short distances, and nerves that go great distances. For example, your optic nerve goes a very short distance, from your brain to your eyes. It gathers the information from your retina and sends it back to the vision center of your brain, which then interprets the data. That is how you understand what you see. All of your cranial nerves stop somewhere interesting in your body and relay the information that is there back to the brain. Without these cranial nerves, we wouldn't be able to understand what we see, hear, feel, smell, or taste.

What Is the Vagus Nerve?

The nerve that wanders the most, from the brain to the lower body, is the vagus nerve. In fact, its very name means 'wandering' since it travels from the brain all the way down to the colon. It is the longest nerve that is a part of your autonomic nervous system. The wandering vagus nerve is your connection between your brain and how your body feels. When people tell you to "listen to your body" or "follow your gut," they're basically telling you to listen to and follow your vagus nerve. But that doesn't flow off the tongue quite as easily. Your vagus nerve is incredibly insightful! In an infinite loop, the vagus nerve interprets your environment and sends signals to your organs to act in a specific way. Likewise, your body's reaction can then tell the vagus nerve what is happening in your environment, which causes it to react again. And so on and so on in a never-ending loop. Your vagus nerve is vitally important to understand your own mental and physical well-being, and understanding how and why your body reacts a certain way in a specific environment.

What Does It Do?

Like all good things, the vagus nerve is multipurpose. While the optic nerve only handles one thing (interpreting sight), the vagus nerve juggles so many different aspects of your body. The most important thing it does is connect your brain's understanding of envronment and experiences and translate that into responses from your major organs like your heart, lungs, and gastric system. It impacts all aspects of how you respond to different stimuli. Let's look at some examples.

On any given Friday or Saturday night, you're probably going to go out with friends. For this example, imagine that these people are your close friends, not just acquaintances or the new guy from work. When you first walk into the restaurant or your friends' home, your body immediately starts to change. Your heart rate slows, and your breathing deepens. You feel warm, comfortable, and can easily understand your friends' facial expressions. You're fully engaged with what is happening and respond to their actions with similar ones. Your body language is more open and you feel a sense of freedom. Your facial expressions probably match the facial expressions of your friends, and you generally feel safe. At this moment, if you take the time to listen to your body, you'll be aware of all of these reactions. Your body's response to this environment and these people is all due to your vagus nerve. It regulated your heart rate, created the feeling of safety, helped you become socially engaged by understanding and reflecting the emotions around you, and helped your body relax. The experience of being with loving, safe people resulted in your vagus nerve creating loving, safe reactions in your body.

When you say goodbye to your friends and start your long walk home in the dark, your body will start going through different reactions. The warmth that you felt before will begin to dissipate, and as the loneliness seeps in, your heart rate will increase. On a dark, lonely walk home, you may become hyper-focused to what's around you. If you hear someone walking behind you, your breathing may increase, your heart rate may increase, and you may start feeling a little twitchy. Depending on your past experiences, the area you live in, or even depending on the experiences of others like you, your body may slowly start to go into flight or fight response if you hear someone walking behind you. You may feel anxious, and your palms may start to sweat. Every horror movie or story you've ever heard before will start to replay in your head as you continue walking home. Every shadow may seem to jump out at you, and every footstep behind you may seem infinitely louder. All of this is your vagus nerve reacting to your past experiences and connecting with your current environment. It's warning you of danger, whether there is an actual danger or not. Your sweaty palms, rapid heartbeat, and accelerated breathing are not because of your vagus nerve's actions but are rather because of its inaction. Your vagus nerve helps you feel calm and safe, so in situations where you might feel like you're in danger, your vagus nerve responds with, "Why yes, you *are* in danger, so I won't stop your body's necessary reaction." Essentially, your vagus nerve decides to sit back with some popcorn and see what comes out of the situation, rather than trying to calm you down. While it's an automatic response, there are things you can do to restore calm and change your vagal response.

This scenario is one of mild stress, but it can quickly become severe stress if you've had previous, terrifying experiences in the dark. Your vagus response can be completely disengaged if your brain and body feel like they're about to experience trauma. This is the fight, flight, or freeze response of your body. We'll discuss this response more within this chapter and later within the book.

From the examples above, we can see that your vagus nerve affects your physiology or your body's responses. We can also see that it can affect your mental responses too. Let's take a closer look at how the vagus nerve works with your body and mind.

Effects on physiology

The wandering vagus nerve touches many of your major organs, and because of this, it controls a lot of sensory and motor actions for those organs. The major systems that the vagus nerve affects are your cardiovascular system, your digestive system, and your respiratory system.

Your cardiovascular system is like a mail sorting system. Except, of course, it's a life or death mail sorting system. It deals with how your blood gets around your body, and how your blood delivers packages of necessary items like oxygen, carbon dioxide, and nutrients to each cell. The vagus nerve deals with your heart and blood pressure, two things that are critical to life and your cardiovascular system. In the examples mentioned earlier, you may have noticed some physical effects for each of the situations. There were signs like a slowed heartbeat while feeling safe. During signs of distress, there were opposite actions like increased heart rate. These differences are because of how your vagus nerve affects your heart. The vagus nerve can slow down your heart rate and lower your blood pressure. So in times of safety, your vagus nerve is actively keeping you calm and your heart rate low. In times of perceived danger, your vagus nerve steps back and lets your body increase your heart rate. In your cardiovascular system, your vagus nerve is responsible for keeping things low and steady.

Your vagus nerve is also closely connected with your digestive system. The moment you eat food, you are using your digestive system. From your esophagus, down through your stomach and liver, and ending at your colon, your digestive system is responsible for processing the food you eat, and turning them into nutrients for your body or waste to be discarded. Your vagus nerve touches many parts of your digestive system. It connects with your stomach and regulates the release of digestive juices that break down your food. It also regulates the contraction of muscles to move food along and connects with your liver and pancreas to release hormones to help with the nutrient use. Additionally, your vagus nerve helps signal to your brain when you are still hungry and when you are full.

If you're familiar with watching or even reading crime dramas, then you'll probably remember the multiple detectives saying, "I know there's no evidence, but I'm following my gut," or something similar. Everyone in the show roles their eyes until the detective is proven right, and their gut is vindicated. You've probably also experienced something. You might call it intuition, or following your own gut when making decisions. But did you know this is an actual thing? Following your gut is absolutely correct! Your gut literally tells your brain things that influence your emotions based on the environment (Klarer et al., 2014). And the way it gets its message across is with the vagus nerve. Your gut is a strange, sensory organ and is very intimately connected with the outside world and the inside body. Because of this connection, your gut, or rather your gut microbiota, can actually detect and sense changes, and it sends these warnings to your brain via the vagus nerve. Your brain's reaction might be one of fear, anxiety, relaxation, or a changed mood. Either way, your gut and your vagus nerve work together to help you make emotional decisions.

The final system that your vagus nerve affects is your respiratory system. This is your body's way of getting oxygen to your cells and includes your obvious organs, the lungs. The vagus nerve helps your lungs regulate each breath. This means it helps determine the timing of your inhales and exhales and how much you are inhaling and exhaling. In the examples before, there were two different types of breathing pattern experiences. The first was slow, deep breathing when you are in a safe place with safe people. The second was quick, shallow breathing when you are in a questionably unsafe environment. This is your vagus nerve responding to the two different environments. In the safe one, it is telling your body to relax. But in the unsafe environment, your vagus nerve disengages and lets your adrenaline and cortisol take care of everything.

Your vagus nerve is critical in many of your body's systems, but there are other ways that it affects your physiology:

- It activates the pharynx and larynx to help with swallowing and speaking.

- It's connected to your gag reflex, which is why if you don't have one, it could be a sign of a malfunctioning vagus nerve.

- It's responsible for reactions like sneezing, coughing, and vomiting.

- It can suppress inflammation in various areas of your body by controlling the release of anti-inflammatory chemicals.

If your vagus nerve isn't fully functioning, then you might have difficulty in all of these areas. You may have cardiac arrhythmias or an inconsistent heart rate. Your blood pressure may also be inconsistent, being too low or too high. You may faint a lot or more frequently because of the changes in your heart rate and blood pressure. You may have some digestive issues with bloating, pain, vomiting, or nausea. And finally, you may see changes in your voice quality or even your ability to speak at all.

Effects on mental health

The effects that your vagus nerve has on your mental health are closely related to how it works within the autonomic nervous system. Your autonomic nervous system controls your automatic, unconscious bodily actions. Within the autonomic nervous system are three parts: the enteric, sympathetic, and parasympathetic systems. For this discussion, we'll focus on the sympathetic and parasympathetic systems. These two parts of the autonomic nervous system work together in perfect balance. They provide your body with key responses to different environments. The sympathetic nervous system is your 'flight-fight-freeze' response system and your parasympathetic is your 'rest and digest' system. Both of these systems can affect your mental health and well-being.

The 'flight-fight-freeze' response is your sympathetic nervous system's response to terrifying or stressful experiences. Fight and flight often occur together. In this situation, you may feel a certain amount of helplessness and stress. There can be a lot of fear and anxiety involved. Your physiology changes, and your body starts preparing to escape the situation. Our lives are already fairly stressful and often, the sympathetic nervous system being overactive can lead to increased anxiety or depression. In the freeze response, everything is increased and the anxiety becomes extreme. This usually comes around because of trauma and can result in PTSD with recurrent freeze states in non-dangerous situations. This is where your vagus nerve comes in.

Your vagus nerve is the main nerve for the parasympathetic nervous system and is all about calming you down. The parasympathetic nervous system is called the 'rest and digest' system for a reason. When your vagus nerve is functioning correctly, your body will be calm and in a state of rest. When your sympathetic nervous system engages, your parasympathetic system and vagus nerve should also activate to help calm you down again once you're safe. However, if this doesn't happen, then you remain in a state of anxiety, which leads to difficulty with mental health and well-being. Later in this book, we'll explore some struggles we all go through and how we can activate our vagus nerve and parasympathetic system to bring our body back to a state of calm.

One thing that can be very surprising is that even minor fears can be interpreted as an actual danger by your vagus nerve, resulting in disengagement. That's why your heart races during a presentation or job interview. It's why you start to sweat or feel anxiety in situations that are not life-threatening. This is your sympathetic nervous system activating and your vagus nerve refusing to engage. In these situations, you can always try to 'restart' your vagus nerve to help you calm down. This will be discussed in our chapter on additional techniques.

Here is a chart that spells out our physical and mental reactions to the sympathetic nervous system in comparison to when our vagus nerve is engaged in the parasympathetic nervous system. This chart has been adapted from Babette Rothschild's chart in *The Body Remembers, Vol. 2* (2016).

	Rest and Digest (Parasympathetic)	Active (Beginning of Sympathetic)	Fight/Flight (Sympathetic)	Freeze (Sympathetic)
Situation	Safe, calm, relaxed	Alert to environment	Danger	Threat to life
Cardiovascular State	Heart rate and blood pressure are normal	Increasing heart rate and blood pressure	Fast, strong heart rate, and high blood pressure	Very fast heart rate and blood pressure is very high
Digestive State	Normal or increased	Decreased digestion	Digestion stops entirely	Digestion stops and the bowels and bladder release
Respiratory State	Breathing is normal and steady	Increasing breathing with breaths becoming shallower	Quick and shallow breaths	Very quick breaths with little air being inhaled

Social State	Safe and willing to connect with others	Probably willing to connect with others	Focused more on the environment and less on possible social connections	There is no awareness of others or self; unlikely for social engagement
Emotional State	Calm, relaxed, feeling love or sexual arousal	Anxiety, anger, excitement, shame	Fear or rage	Terror or even disassociation from the experience

Adapted from Rothschild, 2016.

From this chart, we can see how the parasympathetic system is very different from the sympathetic one. When the vagus nerve is activated, it doesn't matter what state you are currently in, it will start to calm you down. However, there can be one negative. If you are in a 'freeze' state, and there doesn't seem to be an end to the threat, your body can activate the parasympathetic system in order to prepare for death. When this happens, you start to lose awareness of everything and completely disassociate from the experience. Your heart rate and breathing rate drop to dangerously low levels as your vagus nerve prepares your body to escape the situation in the only way it can. This only happens in periods of extreme trauma or reliving/rethinking about extreme trauma.

Your sympathetic nervous system and your outside experiences can all influence your mental health for the negative. If in a place where you finally feel safe and calm, your vagus nerve can be activated to bring you back to a state of calmness and relaxation.

Since the vagus nerve is so important, it's easy to become really worried about its functionality. If you're a little anxious to begin with, your brain might be screaming at you, "What if our vagus nerve isn't functional?!?" Cue horror movie soundtrack. However, you don't have to panic. While you won't be able to determine functionality at home, your doctor can. Even if you have a perfectly functional or a malfunctioning vagus nerve, there are a lot of things you can do to help regain or improve functionality. If your vagus nerve is not functioning well, your doctor may give you a device for external stimulation of the nerve. Or they may recommend a more invasive, pace-maker like device for stimulating the nerve. There are also some non-invasive, non-medical treatments that can help, which we'll discuss in this book.

To conclude this chapter, what the vagus nerve does is critically important to functionality. Whether or not it's functioning well can affect how you respond to regular, everyday stimuli. In general, the vagus nerve and its response are fairly stable throughout your adult life, but you can always improve functionality. You can take actions that can hack your vagus nerve by using your body to send different messages to your brain and improve your vagus nerve functionality. In the following chapters, we'll explore more about the vagus nerve and how/why it affects us so much. We'll also look at specific struggles that we all go through, and how we can learn to send a different message through our vagus nerve to handle our experiences and heal ourselves.

Chapter 2:
Fundamentals of Polyvagal Theory

Thus far in the book, I've talked about the vagus nerve as one single nerve that helps you calm down during times of safety. While this is true, the vagus nerve is actually two branches of nerves, and each branch has a separate and unique reaction to the environment. The two branches are the ventral vagus and the dorsal vagus.

Steven Porges was one of the first researchers to look into these two sides of the vagus nerve and define them. This theory is called the Polyvagal Theory, relating to the two branches of the vagus nerve and their functions. According to this theory, the two branches of the vagus nerve work to calm the body in two very distinct ways. The ventral vagus helps us remain calm in safe environments. The dorsal vagus causes us to shut down (also known as freeze, faint, or mental collapse) during a traumatic experience.

The ventral vagus connects to the upper part of our body. It is our social engagement center. When this branch of the vagus nerve is activated, we are ready to engage with others. It is what keeps us in a calm state and ready to connect with our tribe. I don't use this word 'tribe' lightly. I don't just mean the people close to you, but our communities at large. Our brains are made for being part of a group, not for being individual. Because of this, we mirror and learn from those around us and know from their facial expressions and body language what they are trying to communicate. Everything that we do helps establish our tribe and our connection or disconnection to it. Our ventral vagus nerve is essential in this. It causes us to physically respond to people around us by manipulating our facial muscles to create expressions, modulating our vocal tone to soothe others, and filtering out background noises so that we can better understand one another. When we read an exciting book and feel the swoop in our bellies as something happens, that's our ventral vagus nerve. When we watch a football game and stand up and cheer even though we're not physically at the game, that's our ventral vagus nerve. When we watch a movie that brings us to tears, that's our ventral vagus nerve. All of it is engagement with a community and our tribe.

Our ventral vagus nerve, which is the calming center of our parasympathetic nervous system, responds to the environment around us by looking for social cues from others. When someone acts kindly to us or has a soothing tone, you may notice how your body relaxes and calms down. When someone is strident and loud, your body may react negatively by tensing your muscles. From the smallest social cues, our brains can send signals to the ventral vagus to let us know if we are in danger or are safe. The quirk of someone's lips, the angle of their neck, or the arch of their brow can give us key indications of our safety. We do all of this unconsciously. When we receive messages of safety, our vagus nerve gives us physical feelings of safety, relaxation, and feeling restored.

However, if the message we receive is one of threat, then our body starts to change. Our first response is looking for social engagement. Our eyes will widen, our voice will change to one that's more strident, and we'll give off physical expressions showing distress. For example, we can often tell when someone is about to cry or go into an angry outburst by the simplest of movements in their facial expressions. We often respond to this by trying to comfort or diffuse the situation. This is the body's social engagement system trying to find help from others to comfort or diffuse. But if there isn't help from others, then our body starts to activate the sympathetic nervous system and puts us into survivor mode. We go into fight or flight. If this fails or our body believes that we can't get away from the experience, it activates our dorsal vagus nerve. The dorsal vagus nerve immediately puts us into a freeze or collapse state.

The activation of the dorsal vagus nerve results in drastic physical changes. We become disengaged socially, unable to understand the emotional stimuli from others. Our heart rate drops, and we can literally feel as though our heart drops in our body. That visceral feeling is your dorsal vagus nerve. As it continues to activate, our gut stops digesting and we may unconsciously empty our gut. When people soil themselves in times of extreme fear, it's done without their awareness and is activated by the dorsal vagus nerve. Our very awareness shuts down when the dorsal vagus is activated. This, more than even fight or flight, is the first response that people have when something absolutely terrifies them.

All of these systems can play a role in understanding anxiety, trauma responses, and depression. If we know that this is how the body responds to situations, then we can take the time to learn how to activate the ventral vagus nerve to get us back into a state of calm and a place of social engagement. The polyvagal theory suggests that to get out of the freeze state and reactivate the ventral vagus nerve, we need to be engaged differently. Doing deep breathing with slow exhales can help. Doing a repetitive activity like playing catch or rolling a ball can also help by moving our bodies out of freeze and back into a state of calm. In the next few chapters, we'll look at some challenges to our well-being and how to activate the ventral vagus to help us feel calm in times when we are struggling with anxiety, trauma, depression, stress, and more.

Chapter 3:
Vagus Nerve and Anxiety

While a lot of people like to say that they don't experience anxiety, we actually all experience it at one point or another. It just takes different forms and has different levels of severity. Whenever you have a worry or fear, you're feeling anxiety. Since we all worry, we all have anxiety! There is a difference between just regular everyday anxiety and an anxiety disorder. In this chapter, we'll talk about both and how you can activate the vagus nerve to help handle different situations.

General anxiety can occur in any situation where you feel insecure or worried. A common example is having to give a presentation in front of a crowd. Let's say your boss rushes into your office and tells you that some important clients came for an impromptu meeting and you have to give them a presentation now. And that means right now! That feeling you get in your chest the moment your boss rushes in is anxiety. Your boss is probably feeling anxiety as they rush into your office. Once you go into the meeting room, and you start to give your presentation, your anxiety may worsen. You may feel like your heart is racing, and you might start sweating. Your hands could start the dreaded presentation tremble, making your notes wave in the air like a red flag in front of a bull. You may even start to stutter, depending on how nervous you are. All of this is an anxiety response, and it's represented by the beginning of your sympathetic nervous system activating.

If presentations don't make you nervous, then think about other times. Maybe when you found you didn't have enough money in your bank account or when you learned that a loved one was sick. That sudden drop in your stomach and the beginning of panic, all of that is anxiety. However, both of these situations are mild examples of general anxiety. If your anxiety is something that affects you daily, interferes with your life, and causes you significant distress, then you're moving away from general anxiety into an anxiety disorder.

When experiencing an anxiety disorder, your sympathetic nervous system may be more active for longer, and your vagus nerve may be inactive or not willing to engage because it perceives you as being in actual danger when you're not. There are so many different types of anxiety disorders that activate the sympathetic nervous system with reduced responses from the vagus nerve. In adults, the most well-known types of anxiety disorders are social anxiety disorder, panic disorder, and generalized anxiety disorder.

Social Anxiety

Social anxiety can be fairly common. If you're nervous about giving presentations or going to situations with new people, then you may have some social anxiety. However, social anxiety disorder is more severe and usually results in a person completely avoiding situations where they'll have strangers around them. In the U.S., about 7% of the population experiences social anxiety disorder, and as people get older, that number decreases to less than 5% of older adults experiencing social anxiety disorder (APA, 2013). Social anxiety disorder is usually marked by a fear of being critically observed by others, like in social situations where you meet new people or when you have to give a performance. It's all about the fear of people having a negative perception of the person with the disorder. So, social situations tend to provoke anxious thoughts and fears and result in the person trying to avoid the situation or stay in the situation while feeling intense fear. This goes on for a long time, usually more than 6 months, before it's categorized as a disorder. It's important to note that having fear when giving a presentation can be normal. But having fear that goes way beyond what the situation calls for is when it becomes an anxiety disorder.

Having social anxiety disorder can lead to a lot of negative changes in your life. In general, if you're experiencing social anxiety disorder, you'll do everything in your power to avoid social situations. This means that you might choose to stay at home constantly, rather than going out. This can affect your relationships and especially your friendships. It could also impair your ability to care for your children or elderly parents, especially if you can't bring them out to the doctor's office, pharmacy, or school. Social anxiety isn't the fear of leaving home, but the fear of facing negative judgment from others. So the activities associated with being a parent or caregiver can feel overwhelming.

Many people with social anxiety also struggle with work. Starting from a young age, those with social anxiety are more likely to drop out of school due to social pressures. They may want to have a job like a high-powered businessman, but then they change their goals to better accommodate their anxiety. They might choose work that doesn't require any engagement with people. Or they may choose to work from home where they won't have to talk to colleagues beyond the computer. This isn't to say that every person who works in a job where they don't see people, or who works from home, has social anxiety. It's just one of the work options for those who do have social anxiety. This can mean putting aside your own dreams and goals because your social anxiety can't help you in many work situations.

To cope with social anxiety, a lot of people resort to either being alone or using substances to engage socially. People with social anxiety might drink a lot before going to a party since drinking feels like it dulls their anxiety. The drawback to this is the potential for alcoholism and the fact that drinking is simply another kind of avoidance. It's not solving the problem, just giving the false impression of helping. To truly cope with social anxiety, you have to be able to face the situation while managing your fear. Activating your vagus nerve can help in social situations and can help you calm down. We'll talk about specific ways of doing this later in this chapter.

Panic Disorder

Nearly 11% of the population in the U.S. experiences panic attacks (APA, 2013). However, only a small portion of that number experience panic attacks regularly and unexpectedly. This is panic disorder. If a person experiences panic attacks in situations that don't normally trigger them, these are called unexpected panic attacks. If they happen multiple times, then that person might have panic disorder. A panic attack is a quick surge of intense fear. It can occur in expected environments or environments where panic attacks have been triggered before or in unexpected environments. A panic attack can be very frightening to experience because of its quick onset. One moment you're okay or alert, and the next moment you're in an immediate state of flight or fight.

During a panic attack, a person will go through the emotional and physical changes from an engaged sympathetic nervous system. They'll feel like their heart is pounding out of their chest or like their heart is beating very rapidly. They'll sweat, tremble, and shake. Their breathing will be short, and they may even feel like they're being smothered or choking. They may have chest pain or feel nauseous. They may feel faint or dizzy, and they may have hot flashes and chills. Finally, they may have some emotional and mental reactions like feeling detached from themselves or from reality. They may feel intense fear that they're going crazy or that they're dying. Overall, it's a terrifying experience as your body and mind hijack your awareness and your parasympathetic nerves (including the vagus) decide to sit back and watch what happens without stepping in until later.

A panic attack doesn't include all of these symptoms all the time. In general, four symptoms mean that it's a full panic attack, and anything less than four is still a panic attack, but not a full one. Panic attacks can feel a lot like a heart attack. So it's easy to confuse them. We've all seen TV shows or read books where someone has a panic attack but thinks it's a heart attack and goes to the hospital. There, they're told that it was just a panic attack, and it's supposed to be a comedic or shameful occurrence. However, in reality, it is actually better to make sure you're not having a heart attack. After all, a heart attack will kill you, while a panic attack won't. So it's better to have a medical professional check you before just assuming it's a panic attack. This may be one of the reasons why those with panic attacks visit medical professionals far more than those with other kinds of anxiety.

Because panic attacks can be so frightening, people with panic disorder are classified by their behavior while they attempt to avoid the panic attacks. Someone with panic disorder will have an overwhelming concern about future panic attacks. They'll also have persistent concerns about their health and want to know if they're sick or not. They may be highly concerned about social judgment while they're having a panic attack. This can result in a fear of embarrassment, similar to that in social anxiety. Finally, they might be very worried about their own mental functioning. This is especially true if someone is having repeated panic attacks that are unexpected and aren't triggered by anything fearful. Having a sudden unexpected panic attack can make people think they're losing their minds, so this becomes a great concern to them.

All of these concerns lead to avoidant behavior. People will do whatever they can to avoid panic attacks. This might include simple things like reorganizing their entire lives so that they don't have to face panic attacks alone or in an unfamiliar environment. In case you couldn't tell, I'm being sarcastic because that's not simple at all. It's a huge change in their lives if they choose this path to avoid panic attacks. Having to ensure that you're always surrounded by loved ones who will care for you in the event of a panic attack can be draining on you and on the person caring for you. It also means that you won't get the chance to meet or be around new people very often. If you have to ensure that each environment is familiar, then you don't get to explore new environments. And in the event that you have to do something like buy groceries from the new grocery store, you may put it off for a long time. Avoidant behavior is very common when it comes to anxiety, but it never helps the situation. If anything, it just sets you up for more anxiety when you're forced into the situation you tried to avoid. Later in this chapter, we'll cover some strategies you can follow to help activate your vagus nerve while experiencing a panic attack, or right before a panic attack if one is expected. Doing this will help you calm down and reduce your fear.

Generalized Anxiety Disorder

We've already discussed that we all experience anxiety. It's an everyday experience, but it usually doesn't interfere with our lives. We can worry about our finances when we have bills to pay, but if these worries are constantly on your mind and interrupt your ability to concentrate on your daily tasks, then it becomes more like a disorder. Generalized anxiety disorder is experienced by about 3% of the adult population in the U.S. (APA, 2013). It's characterized by feeling anxiety nearly every day during a variety of regular events like work or daily chores. The anxiety doesn't have to be about one specific thing. A person can feel anxious about multiple routine circumstances or about potential events like their health or misfortune to their family. It's completely normal to be worried about a sick family member or one who has experienced a recent trauma. However, in generalized anxiety disorder, people worry when there isn't any trigger or reason for the worry.

Because generalized anxiety order and regular anxiety can sound similar, let's discuss the differences. In general, there are three major differences between regular anxiety and generalized anxiety disorder.

- Disordered anxiety interferes with functioning in your life. If you can't concentrate on work or reduce your anxiety enough to take your children to a parent-teacher meeting, then your anxiety is interfering with your life. If you are overly concerned about the thing that makes you anxious, and you change your whole life to avoid that thing, then anxiety is negatively impacting your life. Regular anxiety or worry doesn't do this. You might worry about paying your bills or your child's grades, but these worries can be easily put aside to accomplish other things.

- Disordered anxiety has a longer duration and occurs without any triggers or reasoning. For example, if you're preoccupied with thoughts about your partner being sick, but there isn't any sign or history of illness, then this is anxiety without a reason. If this worry continues for months and distracts you from other things, then it's disordered anxiety. On the other hand, if your partner has been sick regularly or has a history of illness or was recently diagnosed with an illness, then worrying about their health is completely normal. It's even normal to continue worrying once they're better (for a short-time period, anyway). So if you're constantly worried about something that has no trigger or pre-emptive event, then this is disordered anxiety.

- Regular anxiety isn't symptomatic and doesn't include the physical symptoms of generalized anxiety disorder. You might have some anxiety and shift into the 'alert' stage, but with regular anxiety, you won't feel restless or feel like you're on edge. You won't be easily fatigued and have difficulty with concentration. All of these are the physical symptoms of generalized anxiety. On top of this, with generalized anxiety disorder, people often feel significant distress. In everyday anxiety, this distress isn't present (unless the event itself is distressing).

The worry and anxiety associated with general anxiety disorder are usually very difficult to control, and the disorder can strongly interfere with people's lives. If you're spending your whole day worried about your chores list, needless to say, you're not going to be concentrating on other things. In fact, poor concentration is one of the symptoms of generalized anxiety disorder. A person with this disorder will also feel restless, both during the day and perhaps at night, too. They may feel easily fatigued, perhaps because of poor or unsatisfying sleep. They'll feel irritable and quick to anger over the smallest things because those things add to their anxiety. They will have some muscle tension and will perhaps feel sore, trembling, or twitching. They may have an overly exaggerated startle response, maybe screaming or crying when something startles them. A person with generalized anxiety isn't going to experience all of these symptoms at once, but having at least three and having them occur most days within a six-month period means you may be a candidate for that diagnosis.

Unlike the previous two anxiety disorders discussed, generalized anxiety isn't typically associated with a flight or fight response. Instead, generalized anxiety is mostly about the persistence of the intrusive, worrying thoughts, rather than physiological changes. However, this doesn't mean that you can't work to use your vagus nerve and the parasympathetic nervous system to help with dealing with the anxiety. In the next section, we'll discuss specific strategies for dealing with anxiety from everyday anxiety to specific types of anxiety.

Self-Help Strategies for Anxiety

When you're experiencing overwhelming anxiety or a panic attack, you're not exactly concerned with very difficult steps and options. You want relief immediately. With this in mind, this section is divided into two sub-parts. The first are techniques you can use to help you immediately activate your vagus nerve to give you some relief from your anxiety. The second part includes skills to practice that can help you relieve your anxiety in the long-term. Use both of these parts to help with relaxation and reducing how much anxiety you feel day-to-day. Also, keep in mind that while self-help strategies can definitely help, if you are continuing to feel significant distress, talk to your doctor or therapist. They can help you break down the origins of your anxiety and find relief, either through therapy or medicine, preferably both.

Immediate self-help strategies

Activating the parasympathetic nervous system and the vagus nerve can help with handling the immediate effects of anxiety. As mentioned before, your vagus nerve sends signals to your lungs and heart to slow and relax. The vagus nerve is all about feelings of safety, so activating it at a time when you're feeling overwhelmed is an easy way to immediately feel safer and more relaxed. The activities in this section will help with this. All of them will activate your parasympathetic nervous system. Depending on the type of anxiety you're experiencing, some of these techniques will work better than others. It's a good idea to practice these techniques when you are already feeling calm. If you have a handle on the technique during times of peace, it will be easier to draw on them during times of distress.

The first technique is deep breathing with long, slow exhales. Long exhales activate your vagus nerve and also help to reduce your heart rate. To do this technique, place your hands on your stomach. You should feel your stomach expand as you breathe. This means that you're taking a deep breath, rather than a shallow, chest breath. To start, take a breath in for the count of four. Hold it for two counts, and then release it for eight counts. You should do a full exhale to get the most benefits. You'll start to feel a change in your body, and your muscles should start to relax. If the exhale count is too long for you, you can reduce it, but not lower than the count of four. The pattern is 4 counts of breathing in, 2 counts of holding, and 8 counts of breathing out. So 4-2-8. You can adjust it as necessary, just remember to have a long, slow exhale.

Another great technique is grounding. Grounding is all about bringing your awareness back to your present moment immediately. This helps you calm down and relax virtually instantly because it requires you to get out of your thoughts. There are a variety of grounding techniques, but one that is very easy to remember and doesn't require any practice is to use your five senses to ground yourself. Your five senses are seeing, hearing, feeling (touch), smelling, and tasting. So using these five, preferably in this order, can help you ground yourself. To do this, say five things that you see around you. Then list four things you hear, three things you feel, two things you smell, and one thing you taste. An example of this technique is this: I see a plant in front of me, a dog on the floor, my computer screen, the gray curtain, and a watering can. I hear the birds outside, the rumble of the A.C., the ticking of a clock, and the soft music from my computer. I feel the keyboard beneath my fingers, the floor beneath my feet, and the sleeve of my shirt on my arm. I can smell the coffee from my cup and the flowers on the plant. I can taste the coffee I just drank. If this feels too long for you, then simply reduce it by counting your five fingers, one for each sense. So just say one thing you see, hear, touch, smell, and taste, counting off on your fingers.

A technique that is a good option but needs to be prepared a little beforehand is visualization. Visualization has many different meanings depending on your goals. In this case, visualization is about bringing up an image in your mind that can help to calm you in any situation. It's about taking your mind to a safe place that you know intimately well. This place should be calming and comforting. It should be someplace that's easy to bring up. There can be people there, or not, but it has to be one of your most well-loved places. Here's how to do this. Close your eyes and think about your most-loved place. You should picture it in your mind completely. Think about what time it is in this place, why you love it so much, the sights, sounds, and scents that are associated in this space. Think about who is there with you in this space, or if you're alone in the space, then enjoy the solitude. Stay in your visualized space until you feel like your anxiety has released and you feel calmer. Then slowly bring your awareness back to the present moment and location. This technique can be very useful, but it does take a little bit of practice. After all, you have to know ahead of time where you want to go when you visualize. Otherwise, it won't help you when you're having a panic attack or are overwhelmed by anxiety.

When you're feeling particularly distressed, but you're in a safe space, sensory experiences can help to calm you down. You could literally go to your visualization space if it's nearby, but you could also do other things that require you to use a specific sense. Some people like to listen to music when they're feeling anxious. So people put their phones to the side and instead just stare at the clouds in the sky or stop to listen to the noises around them. Many people find immediate calming relief by cuddling with a pet or loved one. All of these options are sensory and require you to focus on your outside experience, rather than your inner turmoil. This can help your mind divert itself from anxious thoughts and instead focus on what you are experiencing in the present moment.

Some people find that talking to their vagus nerve or anxiety helps with feeling calmer. Personalizing these two things which are not real people can help you feel more put together. If you are about to give a big speech to your company and are feeling very anxious, stopping to talk to your anxiety can help you feel more in control. You might say things like, "Back off Anxiety, I'm going to do great. You can't hold me back." If you're talking to your vagus nerve, you might reprimand it for leaving you feeling nervous or welcome it back once you feel calm again. These conversations can help you with feeling calmer because they give you a sense of control. You're controlling your experience, and even better, you're changing your thoughts while reprimanding your anxiety and encouraging your vagus nerve. It can be very useful, but be careful that no one hears you while you speak or they may look at you a little strangely. If you're confident enough, you can explain to them exactly what you're doing and why it's helping. Otherwise, let them believe that they believe and continue moving forward to give your speech.

Each of these techniques activates your parasympathetic nervous system and your vagus nerve. Because they all result in a reduced heart rate and breathing rate, they will provide you with relaxation and relief. However, some of them may not work for you, so find the ones that you're most comfortable with. Deep breathing and grounding are scientifically supported to help nearly everyone, so start from there and move on to other techniques if you want to.

Long-term strategies

It's easy to look at the quick fixes and just stick with them. After all, if you can manage the symptoms, then that's all you need, right? You could just use the techniques above, but they're not going to help you resolve your anxiety. Instead, you need to take additional steps to help you work through your anxiety in the long-term. This is done by working through your anxious thoughts, changing negative perceptions, finding coping skills, and practicing new skills. All of these can help you reduce how much anxiety you experience in your life. It can even help you with managing future situations where stress and anxiety overwhelm you. Continue using your quick fixes, but also look to solve the main issues as well.

In this section, we're going to talk about all the strategies you can use to increase your well-being and reduce your anxiety. You can explore these strategies on your own, but it's a good idea to work with a therapist or a support group to give you the necessary feedback on how the strategies are working for you. If these strategies don't work for you at all, then consider talking to a therapist, who can provide you with individual-specific coping strategies and resolutions.

To start with resolving your anxiety, you need to know how it hits you and what triggers your anxiety response. You can use a variety of worksheets or online websites to help with this, but an easy way to do this is by journaling. When you journal, draw a stick figure that represents you. Then think about the last time that you had an anxiety response. Write down all the ways your body reacts physically. Did your muscles tense up, did your heart rate speed up, or did your breathing become erratic? Knowing how your body reacts can help you know when you're being triggered and when your body is about to respond. Once you do this, draw another stick figure and write down how your body feels when you're in a relaxed state. Draw it out on the stick figure. Knowing this can help you look at ways to help remind you that your anxious state is not your permanent one. It doesn't have to control you all the time.

Another activity to do to help you understand more about your anxiety is to draw a pyramid. Divide it into five parts, with part number 1 at the bottom of the pyramid and part number 5 at the top of the pyramid. Using this, write down situations that make you feel only a little or not anxious in part number 1, then go up the pyramid with situations that make you more and more anxious until you get to number 5. In the number 5 section, list situations that are the most anxiety-inducing for you. This can help you better understand which situations you'll need your immediate techniques in, and also what situations you need to work on the most to reduce your anxiety.

Once you've done this, it's time to consider what exactly causes your anxiety. You might immediately want to go to that chart and say that all those situations cause your anxiety. But in reality, they don't. These situations put you in an anxious state, but they don't cause your anxiety. You cause your anxiety. That sounds really confrontational, so let me explain. Our thoughts are really powerful. They can convince us to believe in our worldview, and once we're convinced by our thoughts, we often don't change. For example, if you know for a 'fact' that dogs are vicious, then no matter what evidence there is to the contrary, it's going to be hard to change your belief. In this example, how do you react to those thoughts? You probably avoid all dogs, thus never giving yourself a chance to be exposed to a kind, sweet dog. In this way, it is our thoughts that create our anxiety.

In general, you can explain your thoughts and their effects by looking at the ABC model. In this model, we have our Activating situation (the specific situation or perceived situation), which then influences our Beliefs (our negative thoughts), and results in Consequences (our behavior, actions, and feelings of anxiety). If our thoughts are negative about a situation, then it impacts how we react to that situation and to the world in general. This can be applied to all types of anxiety. So to combat anxiety in the long-term, you need to re-evaluate your thoughts. This can help give you a perception of control over your anxiety (or panic attacks), change your self-talk, and change your negative perceptions.

Let's look at an example:

Activating Situation	Beliefs (irrational negative thoughts)	Consequences
I'm at a party and some girls in the corner are whispering and laughing. (Social anxiety)	They must be laughing at me! Maybe I have bad breath, or I'm not popular enough. I'm so worthless.	Start feeling extremely anxious, shaky, and possibly choose to avoid all parties in the future so that I don't feel that way again.
I have a panic attack at the mall.	Oh my gosh, why am I like this? What's happening? Everyone is watching! Am I sick? I must be crazy! I'm going to keep having these forever.	Panic attack symptoms get worse and are more likely to happen the more I fear them. I change around my life to ensure that my partner is nearby to help me cope with the panic attacks.
I read an article about meningitis. (Generalized anxiety disorder)	Oh my gosh! What if my kids have meningitis! What if they start to have fevers! I won't be able to live with myself if they get sick! I need to make sure they're constantly safe. I should take them to the doctor, just in case. I need to stop everything right now and go help my sick children.	Stop doing work to do more research about meningitis, continue to feel increasing fear and anxiety about the 'problem,' overly distressed about my kids who are not actually sick, nor are they likely to get sick. I will probably try to do everything in my power to make sure they don't get sick, like withdrawing them from school.

In this example, we can see how the activating events result in irrational beliefs, which then have real consequences, like avoiding future situations or making a bad life decision. Instead, we have to work to reframe thoughts. Reframing our thoughts means being aware of them to begin with, and then questioning their accuracy. For our first thoughts listed above, we might reframe them this way:

Irrational belief 1: They must be laughing at me! Maybe I have bad breath, or I'm not popular enough. I'm so worthless.

Reframe 1a: What evidence do I have that they're laughing at me? Do I hear them talking about me in particular? Is it possible that they're laughing about something else? Oh, I see, they're pointing to their phone as they laugh. Maybe they found a funny tweet. It's not about me. I'm okay, and I will be fine at this party.

Reframe 1b: What are the chances that they're laughing at me? Even if they are, and it does suck to be laughed at, it doesn't change my self-worth. Their opinion doesn't change who I am or what I'm worth. While I'll be sad if they're laughing at me, I'll be okay, and I will not allow them to damage my self-confidence. I'll go to a different area with people I know and love, ignoring those girls in the corner.

The reframe obviously depends on the context, but it's important to actually negate your negative beliefs. If your first belief is irrational, you need to be aware of that and take a moment to stop, breathe, and then reframe your thoughts. If this is hard to do at the moment, do it once you're in a safe space. Make a chart like the one above, with your activating situation in one column, your irrational beliefs in the second column, and the consequences of that belief in the third column. This can help you identify how the beliefs hurt you, but it also gives you a chance to reframe them in our safe space. As you keep reframing, try doing it right after having a negative thought. Keep practicing so that reframing becomes your new normal, and one day, you won't have an irrational belief, but rational ones.

Reframing your thoughts will give you literal control over the situation, which can help you immediately feel calmer and more secure. It's important to practice them often by also choosing to avoid the situations. If you avoid them, you won't have to practice reframing, but you'll also keep having an anxious response to those situations in the future. So take the time to slowly expose yourself to situations where you have the opportunity to reframe your negative thoughts. The whole point is to remain aware of your thoughts without being submerged in them. If you have social anxiety, your small practices might include doing small things like saying good morning or giving a compliment to a coworker. You might increase to saying hi to a stranger. It's up to you to determine which situations will help you practice without giving you full-blown anxiety. A therapist can help you with this by breaking down what causes your anxiety and finding small steps for exposure.

To conclude this chapter, anxiety can change your life and how you function within it. However, you can use immediate techniques like deep breathing and grounding to activate your vagus nerve and reduce your anxiety. But don't stop there. Keep working on reframing your thoughts in order to reduce how much anxiety you'll feel in the future.

Chapter 4:
Vagus Nerve and Trauma

Trauma and anxiety go hand-in-hand. Often, when we experience trauma, we also experience an anxiety response. However, we often keep reexperiencing the traumatic event, which causes us extreme stress. Since trauma causes a stress response, both will be discussed in this chapter. Additionally, in this chapter, we'll discuss trauma as something both connected to and separate from anxiety.

In general, a traumatic experience is one that makes us feel as though our lives are in danger. It can be a threat or something we feel will definitely kill us. A threat of death might be experiencing a hurricane, but a feeling of actual death might be if someone tries to literally kill us or if we feel like we'll die during a natural disaster. Trauma can also include the exposure to injury or sexual violation. All of these events can create a stress response that results in feeling traumatized. A traumatic experience can happen to us, be witnessed, or even simply be heard about from a loved one. Either way, the trauma response can be similar, as if you had experienced it yourself. People who are repeatedly exposed to the details of trauma can also experience a traumatic stress response. For example, police officers can have a traumatic stress response after having to regularly help children that have been abused.

Trauma is a very heavy topic, mostly because of its devastating effects on our bodies and minds. Trauma can change who we are at our core. A lot of people may say "What doesn't kill us, makes us stronger," but this isn't necessarily true in regards to trauma. What doesn't kill us can make us stronger, but it can also make us feel weak, desperate, and hopeless. Did you know that 70% of adults in the U.S. have experienced trauma at some point in their lives, that a woman is raped every 6 minutes, and that 33% of children exposed to something traumatic experience post-traumatic stress disorder (National Council for Community Behavioral Healthcare, n.d.)? These statistics are concerning, and for the people who experience trauma, it can have life-changing effects.

In general, there are three types of responses to trauma right after the traumatic event occurs, and these connect to the levels of arousal from chapters one and two. The first type of response is mental collapse. This type of response results in people fainting, falling unconscious, or being nearly catatonic. The second type of response is feeling frantic. During this response, there may be feelings of panic and an immediate increase in the sympathetic nervous system. A person may feel the same panic for long after they are safe. The final response type is feeling focused. This is the response people may have where they stay calm and in control. They usually try to help others during the traumatic event. It's important to note that there isn't a judgment associated with the trauma response. Your response is automatic and unconscious. It's a combination of how you were raised, your nature, and your past experiences, and thus doesn't have a moral value to it. So don't feel like your response has to be the focused kind, and any other response is demeaning because that simply isn't true. It's simply a matter of how your body reacts, often without your input.

Judgment also shouldn't be made because ultimately, it doesn't matter how you respond during a traumatic event. What matters is how it affects you as you continue your life. A traumatic event may happen once, or it may be recurring. Your reactions can range depending on the circumstances. But once the traumatic event ends, what happens next? Often people can struggle with their lives after trauma. Some feel severe stress all the time and have difficulty connecting with others. Some people can have difficulty controlling themselves and their own minds. Let me give you an example. This example will discuss a car accident in brief and may be triggering to those who have experienced traumatic car accidents, so please skip the example and move to the paragraph after the example if you feel like you may be triggered.

Example: You and your partner are driving down a city street at nighttime. The streetlight far ahead of you is green, and the car ahead of you goes through it. As they go through the intersection, an 18-wheeler suddenly slams into their vehicle after running a red light. Going too fast yourself, you slam into the first vehicle and the truck, and another car slams into you. The result is a four-car accident. You can see the people in the car in front of you, the first car hit. The car is so badly damaged, you can't see much, but you can hear someone screaming. You desperately try to get you and your partner out of your vehicle, but your partner is unresponsive, and you can't get the doors open. Another driver who was involved in the wreck helps you and your partner out of the car, while passersby try to help the family in the first vehicle hit. You later learn that the family in the first car died before they could be rescued.

This scenario shows the three different reactions to the trauma. Of all the people involved, your response is frantic, your partner is collapsed, and the person who helped you out of the vehicle is focused. However, what happens next is important. Because of the accident and the trauma of it, you and your partner go home relatively unscathed but have a hard time calming down. You both feel the same fear you felt before, but now you're in a safe space. To cope with the fear, you might both choose to drink or take something to numb you. Either way, this feeling of fear doesn't dissipate. You may struggle to get into a vehicle again or drive at nighttime. Your partner may become more emotionally withdrawn. You may have kept in touch with the driver who helped you, and they might also be struggling. The trauma you experienced might not result in damage to you, but for many people, it does result in reduced well-being. Trauma can stick with you for months or years after the event has passed, and it can make it difficult for you to continue on with your life the way it was before.

Let's face it, a traumatic experience will change you. Whether that change is big or small is based entirely on your physiology and how you handle the trauma right after the event. For many people, they turn to alcohol or other substances to help them cope with trauma. In the U.S., this is part of our culture. After all, in most TV shows, you see people dealing with their issues by drinking. So drinking might sound like a good idea. However, if you're still having a trauma reaction months later, then drinking can become a serious problem. Those who have experienced trauma have a higher rate of substance abuse. They also have a higher rate of experiencing abuse again in the future or even becoming an abuser themselves. This all goes back to how our bodies react to trauma.

Some of this was discussed in chapters one and two about the autonomic nervous system and how it responds to danger. Unlike anxiety, trauma really is a dangerous situation, so your body responds accordingly. During the event, your ventral vagus starts by changing your facial expressions and tone of voice to get people to help you. You may literally call for help. However, if there is no response, or you don't get help from others based on your expression, then your ventral vagus deactivates and your sympathetic nervous system takes over. It prepares your body to fight its way out of the situation or to flee it. In the example above, you would have been in fight or flight while having a frantic response to the traumatic event. If there is no way to escape, or if your body has previously learned to freeze, then that's exactly what you'll do. Your dorsal vagus will activate, causing you to freeze or go into mental collapse. In the example above, your partner's reaction is that of freeze.

Now here's the thing. After the traumatic event, once you're in a safe space, your body should start to calm down. Your ventral vagus should activate again and help you calm down. However, because of a variety of circumstances, this may not happen. This puts you in a prolonged fight or flight state or prolonged freeze state. It can increase your anxiety and stress in general. Even when you eventually feel calm again (and you will), you may have things that suddenly reactivate your fight or flight unexpectedly. For instance, using the same couple from the example above, let's say that one day you yell at your partner for something, and they quickly find themselves going into the freeze state. Or you may get into a car and automatically go into fight or flight because of your past experience. This is how your body remembers the trauma, and depending on how often trauma is experienced, this sudden shift in physiology during safe times can last for years. It can hamper your social interactions and even what you do in your daily life. So trauma can have long-lasting consequences.

Whether you experience one traumatic event or experience repeated ones, like in the case of abuse, the experience can lead to our brains and autonomic nervous system misinterpreting the information it's given. Trauma can cause our sympathetic nervous system to activate too easily and be triggered even when you're in a safe situation. The smallest things that remind your body of the traumatic experience can result in triggering your sympathetic nervous system. It could be something small like a scent or an emotion on someone's face. It doesn't have to be a big thing that triggers your sympathetic nervous system and deactivates your ventral vagus nerve. However, what can be even more distressing is that your body and brain can see dangerous situations and not activate your sympathetic nervous system. So dangerous situations can cause you not to react, resulting in further trauma. These misfired activations can damage your situational awareness, your understanding of safety, and your relationships, especially with those who don't know what you're going through. Children who have parents that experienced trauma know this. They remember when their parents would overreact to small stimuli or be aggressive when aggression wasn't called for. So trauma can have far-reaching effects in relationships as well as situational awareness.

Trauma can result in fourteen symptoms that can affect your well-being. In general, no matter your response to trauma, you will experience some of these symptoms, but they are often a normal response to trauma. However, if you experience multiple symptoms, then you may be having a prolonged stress response. Here are the fourteen symptoms you may experience after a traumatic event:

1. Memories of the event that are recurrent and intrusive. They may be involuntary memories, occurring when you least expect them or when you're not actively thinking about the event.

2. Dreams that are recurrent and distressing. Again, these may be about the event or the things that happened immediately before or after the event.

3. Flashbacks of the event that are disruptive and occur unexpectedly.

4. Intense distress after being triggered by something that reminds you of the event.

5. Feeling like you don't have positive emotions, and being unable to express positive emotions.

6. A change in your perception of reality.

7. Being unable to remember pieces of the event. Often, our minds will hide parts of the event that were the most distressing to us so we can't remember them.

8. Actively avoiding experiencing memories, feelings, or thoughts about the event.

9. Actively avoiding physical or external reminders about the event. You may avoid the people involved in the event, places where it happened, or activities associated with it. You may even avoid talking about the event altogether.

10. Having poor, unsatisfying sleep. You might often wake up or be unable to fall asleep at all.

11. A change in behavior, resulting in more irritability, even over simple things. This can lead to aggression, either verbal or physical.

12. Hypervigilance. This means trying to be constantly aware of your environment. It can increase your stress levels because it's simply not possible to remain in such a state for a long period of time.

13. Problems with concentrating, especially with concentrating on your next steps after the event.

14. An exaggerated response to being startled. You may feel startled by things that, in the past, wouldn't have bothered you or resulted in a reaction.

It's important to remember that some people don't face all of these negative aspects of trauma. They don't experience lingering effects after a few days, and thus, may not need or want additional help. If, however, you've been experiencing lingering effects from trauma, then consider talking to a therapist or doctor. They can help you with adjusting to your current life and the effects the trauma has on it. They may give you a diagnosis like acute stress disorder or post-traumatic stress disorder (PTSD). Notice how they both have the word 'stress' in them. This is because after experiencing trauma, your body goes through recurrent stress responses. Let's look at these two possible diagnoses below.

Acute stress disorder is the first diagnosis you may receive if you're experiencing lingering effects from the trauma. This diagnosis is only possible 3 days after the traumatic event and up to a month afterward. This is because, for some kinds of trauma, the effects after it are reduced as the days go by. For example, after a devastating hurricane, communities often come together to help one another cope with the trauma of the event, which can help people adjust. So acute stress disorder is only diagnosed in the first month after the event and only after the first few days have passed. To be diagnosed with acute stress disorder, you have to have experienced a traumatic event and experience at least nine of the traumatic symptoms listed above. There also can't be another reason (like a medical disorder) for the traumatic experience.

After one month, the diagnosis of acute stress disorder is no longer valid. However, if the stress response and traumatic symptoms are still occurring, then you may have PTSD. This is a fairly common word associated with trauma. While most people know about PTSD when thinking about war or veterans, PTSD can be experienced by anyone who has experienced trauma. PTSD has many of the same symptoms that were mentioned earlier, but also additional ones like different cognitive functioning and physiological responses. On top of the symptoms already mentioned, there can be a lot of cognitive changes. These include negative thoughts about themselves and of others or the world; negative emotions like persistent fear, anger, shame, or guilt; and distorted beliefs about the event that can cause the victim to blame themselves for events. There can also be reduced interest or participation in activities and reduced social engagement. There can be an increase in self-destructive behavior.

Sometimes PTSD is also connected with dissociative symptoms. These include flashbacks, feeling depersonalization, and derealization. Flashbacks are when you feel like you are reliving the event itself. It can be really small like having a very short period of time where you think you hear or feel the things you did during the event. Or it can be really severe like you're fully there and are completely unaware of your current environment. Depersonalization is feeling like you aren't attached to your body, almost like you were observing your actions without being able to change them. Derealization is feeling like your environment is unreal, distorted, or dreamlike. This can, obviously, be very distressing to people and can result in putting you into a constant state of anxiety and stress.

Because of how distressing trauma can be, it's important to take the time to activate your ventral vagus immediately after the traumatic event once you're safe. This can help with coping. Additionally, as the days go by, or even if you experience a prolonged stress response for months, you can take action to help activate your vagus nerve and relieve some of your traumatic symptoms. Before we continue with the self-help strategies, remember, it's always a good idea to talk to your therapist or doctor when it comes to trauma, since trauma can have a drastic effect on your life and well-being.

Self-Help Strategies for Trauma

Just like for the chapter on anxiety, this section is divided into two parts: immediate self-help strategies and long-term self-help strategies. Before we get into them, I want to discuss the importance of social support for treating trauma. Trauma itself, and its effects on our responses to the environment and people can severely impact our social engagement since we're constantly put into a state of 'survival.' In this state, our ventral vagus nerve isn't activated and we can't nurture those around us. So instead, at that moment, we must rely on others to promote our feelings of safety.

Since we are not individuals as much as a tribe, having social support after a traumatic event is crucial. After all, feeling safe and being safe with other people is probably the most important need for our well-being. So consider your social support. This can be people in your community or culture who can provide you with that safety and well-being. They should be people who you can count on and who will understand where you are coming from. Often, communities band together after a traumatic event and can help each other heal. So consider social resources. If you don't have any, then consider getting a pet. Dogs and horses are two animals that are often used for helping those with PTSD. There are also many programs where you can go and work with horses as part of your healing.

As you're choosing your path to healing a traumatic past, consider your own cultural context. The suggestions coming up are based on generic healing, but often, our cultures have their own take on healing and coping with trauma. So consider some cultural aspects of trauma that can help you. Depending on your culture, there can be traditional healing methods that can help. Often, these methods are really well chosen and can definitely help. It's important that you choose your healing methods either based on your own culture or on scientific backing. Taking another culture's healing methods might work for you, but there's really no guarantee if you're not closely connected to that culture. Our beliefs impact our healing, so choose healing methods that align with your personal beliefs. If you choose to work with a therapist, then find one who will respect your cultural beliefs and will help you discuss trauma in that context.

One last thing about these strategies is that some may or may not work for you based on your traumatic experience. Some people have a hard time focusing on their body or creating body awareness after trauma happens, so if you choose to practice these, do so in a safe place and pay attention to how you react to the exercises. If you're concerned about the possibility of body awareness triggering you, then choose exercises that don't require it. The grounding exercise, meditation, and working with animals don't require body awareness, at least not the way they're explained in this chapter. Choose only the activities that actually bring you relief, and find other alternatives if none bring you relief.

Immediate self-help strategies

The strategies in this part will work to help you activate your vagus nerve and calm your stress responses. You can use these techniques in the aftermath of trauma once you are safe but are still keyed up. You can also use them if you feel like you are dissociating from your reality or are having a flashback. Really, anytime that you feel your sympathetic nervous system activates, you can use these techniques to calm down, as long as you are in a safe space. Practice these activities when you feel safe and in control before trying them when you feel distressed. Finally, let your loved ones know these activities so that they can help you with them in the event that you are in a frozen state where you have completely dissociated from the present moment. The activities in this section are progressive muscle relaxation, grounding, meditation, and physical activity. They can all be done alone or with the help of your social support system.

Progressive muscle relaxation sounds a little weird, but I promise it works. This type of muscle relaxation requires you to focus on muscles in specific areas of your body, usually moving from your hands to your head, then down to your toes. You can, of course, change the pattern as you wish. To do progressive muscle relaxation, you are going to tense your muscles in the specific area of your body, holding for about 5 seconds before releasing all at once. Then take a couple of seconds to be aware of the difference in your body. You should tense as you breathe in, and release as you breathe out. Then continue to the next area to tense and relax.

You can do this anywhere with just tensing your arms and legs, or if you want to do a full-body progression, you should be in an area that is safe and peaceful. Here's an example of one you can do anywhere:

- Starting from your fingers, tense your fingers and hold for 5 seconds.
- Release all at once.
- Be aware of how your fingers feel.
- Move up to your hands. Clench them and hold for 5 seconds.
- Release all at once.
- Bring awareness to your hands.

- Move up to your forearms. Tense the muscles there and hold for 5 seconds.
- Release all at once.
- Bring awareness to your forearms.
- Move up to your upper arms. Tense the muscles there and hold for 5 seconds.
- Release all at once.
- Bring awareness to your upper arms.
- Move up to your shoulders. Tense the muscles there and hold for 5 seconds.
- Release all at once.
- Bring awareness to your shoulders.

At this point, you can reverse directions if you want to and move back to your fingers. If you want to continue the exercise, move up to your face starting with your forehead, down to your eyes, then your cheeks, lips, and neck. Then continue down until you reach your toes.

Once you're finished with the relaxation, the important thing is to bring awareness to how your body feels. Then take a few breaths in with deep exhales to continue activating your vagus nerve.

Using grounding is another great technique to help you when you are experiencing a stress response, flashback, or discomfort from traumatic memories. You can follow the grounding strategy in the chapter on anxiety, but here is another option. In this type of grounding, you are looking at color and shape instead of focusing on the five senses. It's a very quick way to bring your awareness back to the present moment and out of a flashback if you're experiencing one. As you ground yourself, try to even out your breathing, and if possible, start a breathing pattern with longer exhales. Here is the exercise:

- Look at the floor beneath your feet. What color is the floor? What is it made of?

- Look at the wall. What color is it? What shapes are on the wall? What other colors (if there are pictures etc.) are there?

- Look back at the floor. What color are your shoes? What color is the floor again? What size are your shoes? Remember where you are right now.

- If you can, take 10 deep breaths with long exhales.

This grounding exercise uses your external awareness to bring you back to the present moment. Take time to categorize what you see to help bring you out of a flashback or dissociation. Your friends and family members can help you with this if you can't clear your mind to do it yourself. Have them ask you those questions, reframing from the one about "where are you right now" since that might make you go back into the flashback. Instead, focus on what is around you, focusing on color, shape, size, etc.

Mindfulness meditation is similar to grounding, in the sense that it asks you to focus on the present moment. It's another great technique to use, but can be difficult if you're using it for the first time, especially if you've experienced trauma. In general, mindfulness meditation requires you to explore your inner world. However, this can cause your traumatic symptoms to increase and activate your sympathetic nervous system. Since that isn't what we want, let's change the mindfulness from internal to external. Additionally, once you've set your stage for mindfulness, ensure that you follow a set pattern so you know exactly what to do when you need to meditate. Mediations can be long or short depending on what you need. Since here, I'll provide two meditation scripts. One is for your external observations, and one is for recollecting positive memories. Depending on your trauma experience, they may not work for you, so proceed with caution. If they don't work, take the time to find something you can do as an alternative.

Nature Meditation Script
1. Take a moment to find a peaceful area, preferably outside. A park or garden can be a good choice. Make

sure that you are comfortable, either sitting or lying down.

2. Once you are comfortable, take a deep breath in and let it out.

3. Look around you. What do you see? Perhaps some animals, maybe a few insects. Take a moment to categorize them. What do they look like? If your mind wanders, gently bring it back to what you are seeing.

4. Take a moment to breathe in and out deeply if you can. What do you smell in the air? If your mind wanders, gently bring it back to what you see or smell.

5. Take another deep breath in, releasing it gently. What do you hear? Take a moment to look for what is making each sound. Categorize them. Are you hearing birds or the wind in the trees? If your mind wanders, gently bring it back to what you see, smell, or hear.

6. Continue as you see fit.

7. When you are ready to end the meditation, take a deep breath in, releasing it gently. Then bring your awareness slowly back to yourself.

Positive Memories Script

1. Take a moment to find a peaceful area. Make sure that you are comfortable, either sitting or lying down.

2. Once you are comfortable, take a deep breath in and let it out.

3. Think about a time or person that made you feel happiness, peace, or safety.

4. What was happening in that memory? How did you feel and what emotions did you experience? Recollect the memory. Try to picture it in its entirety.

5. Take a deep breath in and gently release it. Continue going through the memory.

6. If your mind wanders, gently bring it back to your positive memory.

7. When you are ready to end the meditation, take a deep breath in, releasing it gently. Then bring your awareness slowly back to yourself.

The positive memory script can not only provide you with some relaxation but can also help you find physical things that can help calm you as well. For example, if you remember eating ice cream with your loved ones, then maybe eating ice cream could also calm you when you're feeling stressed. If your memory is about the kindness someone showed you, then perhaps further kindness (from yourself to yourself or from yourself to others) would help you.

The final strategy for this section requires physical activity. Often times, if we are in a state of fight, flight, or freeze, something that is physical and repetitive can help us out. A negative coping skill that involves this is when people cut themselves to help them calm their minds. Instead of cutting, try a different physical activity that has a lower likelihood of hurting you. A good repetitive activity is simply walking and counting your steps. You could also play catch or roll a ball into the wall so it rolls back to you. Yoga is an option, but since this brings body awareness, it might not be right for everyone. If you want something more active, then try running or biking. Hiking can also be a good option. If you can't leave your current environment, then consider carrying around a pebble or shell with you. Use your hands to manipulate the object, which can help you get out of your head and back into your present moment.

Physical activities are also a great option because they can create social engagement, which we already established is critically important. If your loved ones are aware of what you're going through, they can use physical activities to help you if they see that you're in a fight, flight, freeze state. They can roll a ball to you until you start to focus on it. The movement can help someone experiencing a flashback focus on the here and now. Just ensure that your family doesn't touch you when they try to engage you. By including social interactions as part of the physical activity, it can activate your ventral vagus nerve and help reduce your sympathetic nervous system's reactions.

All of these options for immediate help can aid you when you're feeling overwhelmed by your memories. They can put your brain into a safer mindset and help activate your vagus nerve to reinforce the feelings of safety. These activities can also help you with your stress reactions or when your body misinterprets something as being unsafe. Of course, you first have to be aware that your body has activated its sympathetic nervous system. Your family and loved ones can help you with this, as they'll often become aware of it based on your actions. If they're prepared, they can help bring you back into the present moment with these activities.

Long-term coping strategies

It's important to work through your trauma experience to gain the most benefit for your life. Trauma can be resolved, so there is always hope that you won't have to struggle with traumatic stress responses for all of your life. In this section, we'll discuss some options that can help you cope with trauma, but some won't necessarily resolve it; they'll just help you heal from its immediate and long-term effects. These coping skills can help you manage your symptoms and start your healing process. The first is reiterating what has been mentioned before: the importance of having a supportive network.

Many people who have experienced trauma gain a lot of benefit from having a supportive network. This is beyond having your family around you. Instead, a supportive network is a network of people who have also been in the same place as you. Groups like this can help you understand more about why your body and mind are reacting the way they do. Groups can also provide each other services like sharing coping skills that worked for the individuals and providing feedback when things didn't work. Groups are also great for offering life advice. Often, after experiencing trauma, our lives and relationships change. Support groups can provide you with ideas on what has and what hasn't worked for them. They can also provide you with options if you need to find a new safe place to live. Essentially, a supportive group network can give you the social network you need to heal, while also providing you with valuable resources for healing.

In addition to supportive networks, working with a therapist is also recommended. Of course, this depends on your cultural take on therapists, but for the most part, working with one can help you with your mental well-being. If you choose to work with a therapist, find one who is experienced in working with trauma. Unfortunately, many therapists and psychologists are not trained in how to deal with trauma, which means they may not provide you with any benefit. Choose to work with therapists who are experienced in dealing with traumatic responses and who take a humanist perspective, focusing on you as an individual rather than just focusing on generic healing. A good therapist can often be found online using networks like the American Psychological Association (APA) and the American Counseling Association (ACA). Your support group can also recommend therapists or may even be led by one.

If you're at the point in your traumatic recovery where you really don't want to deal with people, then consider getting a pet to help you. Pets can provide your brain with the same emotional support as people can. Of course, pets don't talk back, but they can provide you with comfort and safety, thus activating your ventral vagus nerve to calm you and keep you feeling safe. If you're interested, you can always get a therapy dog, or even a therapy pony, to help with your emotions and stress response. Animals are a fantastic alternative if you don't have a social network that you can trust or feel safe in. Pets can provide you with what you need to feel safe.

Many times, those who experience trauma find support in their spiritual or religious beliefs. If you are someone who has a spiritual belief, then use that to help you heal. Many people find prayer helpful when dealing with struggles, so if you're religious, then take advantage of this type of healing and coping. Additionally, you can find a strong supportive network in spiritual and religious groups. Often, and depending on the spiritual following or religion, you can find a lot of people who are willing to help you with your struggles and support you as you heal. So take advantage of that! Finally, many people find that their spiritual or religious beliefs help give them a sense of hope. It gives them a strong belief that things will get better and that life will move one. This hope and reassurance can really help with healing from trauma.

To bring this chapter to its conclusion, it is possible to heal from trauma. Learning how your body reacts to the reminders of trauma and then activating your parasympathetic nerves to help calm you are the key factors for coping with traumatic memories. Remember to include your loved ones in your healing process, as social connections can be so incredibly healing after a traumatic experience. In the next chapter, we'll be discussing depression, which is linked to trauma.

Chapter 5:
Vagus Nerve and Depression

Imagine this. You're sitting in a movie theater after watching the ending of *Avengers: End Game.* The lights have slowly come up in the theater, and people are still relatively stunned by the ending of the film. You hear a teenager in the row behind you mutter, "We'll that was depressing." And you agree. You don't feel happy. You might feel sad by the ending and wonder to yourself, what next? However, the moment you leave the theater and go get yourself something to eat, you'll probably notice that your mood is no longer low. It's gone back to its average of contentment, perhaps with some variation as you contemplate the movie you just watched. When people talk about something being depressing, it's usually just a representation of a feeling of sadness or having a low mood. This feeling doesn't stick around for long before the next events happen and your mood changes with them. However, for some people, their low mood doesn't disappear easily. It clings to them far longer than it should and is very hard for them to overcome. This is depression.

Depression is a problem that many people experience in their lives. The level of depression you may feel at any given time really does depend on your environment and the trigger. In general, we can say that people often feel mild depression, moderate depression, or severe depression. Mild depression is manageable and often doesn't affect your social spheres of life too much. Some people call this 'high functioning depression,' meaning that they function well at work and socially as needed, but the moment they're home alone, they're hit by the freight train of depression again. Moderate depression shows some effect on social functioning, with more serious symptoms. Severe depression has a large number of negative effects on social functioning and is generally considered very distressing and unmanageable. Whether the depression you're feeling is manageable or severe, activating your vagus nerve can help with coping with depression, and medical activation of the vagus nerve can help with severe depression.

There are so many different kinds of depression, but the basic symptoms are often similar; they just change in severity. General depression involves feeling, well, depressed. It involves a melancholy mood or feeling sad or hopeless. Depending on how self-aware you are, you might observe these feelings, or someone else might and they'll point it out to you. Beyond sadness, there might even be a lot of irritability beyond the norm and feeling empty. With these feelings comes possible physiological reactions, like frequent crying spells. Beyond having a low mood, you may also feel like there is very little pleasure to be gained from your regular activities. In fact, you may lose interest in all of your activities. This can cause additional distress, as things that used to bring you joy no longer help.

Physically, depression can bring you a lot of changes. You may lose or gain a lot of weight when you're feeling depressed because your appetite will change. It's not uncommon for someone dealing with depression to not feel hungry during the day. They may not even notice that they haven't eaten in a while. With changes in eating patterns come changes in energy. Often, people who are struggling with depression feel significant fatigue. When we think of depression, we often think of someone curled up in bed refusing to leave it. While this might actually happen, what's more likely to happen is just general exhaustion and not having the energy to do basic things like cooking, leaving the house, or even taking care of personal hygiene. You may even see someone who is depressed being actually slow, as in they move slow, talk slow, and react slowly. All of this is from the lack of energy we feel when we're depressed.

Finally, depression takes a significant toll on our emotions. It can cause us to feel like we are worthless or nothing. It can make us have guilt for situations that we shouldn't feel guilty about.

Worst of all, these negative emotions and other aspects of depression can make us think about death and have recurrent thoughts about death. Dying from depression is all too common as depression is one of the leading risk factors of suicidal thoughts.

After all of this, you might be wondering how depression and the vagus nerve go together. After all, in the case of anxiety and trauma, the trouble is with the sympathetic nervous system being on too long, causing a reduction in the vagus nerve's activation. But what about with depression? When you're depressed, you're not going to feel that same, quick rush of fight or flight response randomly, like you might with trauma and anxiety. So what is it? Well, some researchers think that it has to do with your heart rate patterns, which are controlled by your parasympathetic nervous system and your vagus nerve. They believe that, like with anxiety and trauma, in depression, your sympathetic nervous system is too active, which in turn suppresses your parasympathetic nervous system and decreases your healthy heart rate. All of this can then contribute to feelings of depression. This is all related to vagal tone, which we'll discuss more in a later chapter. Suffice it to say, trying to activate more of your vagus nerve can help with putting your body back in balance, improving your healthy heart rate pattern, and reducing your depression.

Self-Help Strategies for Depression

In the previous two chapters, this section was separated into two parts, short-term and long-term strategies for improving symptoms. This format generally worked because anxiety and trauma can produce situations where you feel like you need help immediately, like when you're having a panic attack or flashback. Depression doesn't really have points like this. So instead of dividing this section into two parts, it's going to be just one part exploring different kinds of self-help strategies for depression. The strategies we'll discuss are reframing cognitive distortions, relaxation techniques, and exercise. We'll also discuss some techniques that may be useful for different kinds of depression.

Cognitive distortions

Since depression can cause a low mood and low self-esteem, when we're depressed, we can feel like the world is out to get us. However, this rarely turns out to be true. These thoughts can create a cycle of negativity that keeps your low mood in effect. These thoughts that we have about how the world feels about us are called cognitive distortions. Cognitive distortions are when we take regular everyday things and assign a negative meaning to them. They create an unconscious bias, and we often keep reiterating the beliefs over and over again. There are many different kinds of cognitive distortions, but here are seven that are often experienced if you have depression or even anxiety.

1. Jumping to conclusions: We often hear this phrase when we misinterpret an event and make a judgment about it. Basically, jumping to conclusions is when we come to our own conclusion about an event without any evidence. Here's an example of jumping to conclusions: You're at a social event and you see someone walk by you while laughing. If you jump to conclusions, you may believe they're laughing at you because you're ridiculous. This is a conclusion that has no evidence but creates a negative bias about yourself.

2. Magnification: When we exaggerate our failures, we are magnifying them, thus creating a suggestion that we are always failures. This can be devastating to anyone who is struggling with self-esteem or depression. For example, if you are generally a good student, getting mostly A's and B's in your class, you may one day fail a quiz. Instead of seeing this as a temporary setback, you may start to think that you are a failure in general. This is a magnification of your small set-back.

3. Minimization: This is right next to magnification, but also the opposite. Minimizing is about reducing the positive in your life or outright dismissing the positive. This means that anytime something good happens to you, you instead put it aside and focus on the negative aspects. For example, let's say that you have been practicing Tae Kwon Do for a long time, and then you win your first competition. Instead of basking in the positive win, you dismiss it and focus on the problems with your form. You may even choose to think that you're mediocre. Another example might be something that happens at work. If you receive praise for a project that was successful, you may dismiss the praise and still consider yourself mediocre at best and barely competent at worst. This is a minimization of your successes. With minimization, you'll never feel confident with accepting that you're more than just average or terrible. Instead, you'll simply choose to keep thinking negatively about yourself.

4. Catastrophizing: When we often exaggerate or minimize our failures and successes, we can easily slip into catastrophizing. This is when we see the worst possible outcome for our actions. When we catastrophize, we may see things as being disastrous, when they clearly aren't. We may also see things as impossible to correct or improve. If we do a project at work and run across a

mistake that we made, it can be easy to beat ourselves up. But if we catastrophize, then we may take our self-flagellation to a whole new level by thinking that the problem is unfixable, we're a failure, and that they'll fire us at any moment. This is probably not true. One small mistake probably won't lead to you being fired, depending on what field you work in. However, if we have this cognitive distortion, then we may be absolutely convinced about our disaster.

5. Overgeneralization: You're probably familiar with this term, but when someone overgeneralizes, they take one instance and make sweeping generalizations based on it. We do this a lot concerning the cultures and races of other people, creating stereotypes. But when it comes to this cognitive distortion, many of the biases are about ourselves and our own abilities. If your job is as a doctor, then you'll probably have a time when you make a misdiagnosis. While this is obviously concerning to yourself and the patient, if you overgeneralize then you may say to yourself that you're stupid or a failure and that you'll never be successful as a doctor. This is very similar to catastrophizing, but it focuses on your career success, and as such, these thoughts can linger for a while. The result is that you'll start doubting your work and may

make future mistakes, thus 'confirming' your generalizations and continuing the cycle of negativity.

6. Filtering: Have you ever been in a relationship and had the person you love to say one thing that was very critical to you? Probably, since arguments and criticism are normal, though infrequent, aspect of relationships. Hopefully, your relationship is good otherwise, with many positive aspects and a lot of love. However, if you choose to focus on that one negative criticism and ignore all the positives surrounding it, then you are choosing to filter out the positives. This can have a profoundly negative effect on your relationships. But beyond this, you can filter in other areas of your social life with the same negative effects.

7. Personalization: You've probably heard people tell you not to take things personally. We usually say this phrase after someone takes an event to heart, even when the intention wasn't to cause the person their negative feelings. Personalization is similar to this. It's when we take something completely arbitrary, and then blame ourselves for it. We take it personally when really, it might not be about us at all. Here's an example. Let's say you walk into your boss's office and she looks really upset. Personalization means that you'll take your boss's appearance and emotions and think that you're the

problem for those emotions. In reality, your boss may have just gotten some bad news or even came into work with a bad mood. You take the blame for something that you have no control over. Personalization can take place in a variety of situations. If you are in a car accident, but it wasn't actually your fault, you may still assign yourself blame and guilt, even though there's no reason to.

Working on cognitive distortions will help you regulate your mood, which, in turn, will help your ventral vagus become a little more active. This can help to relieve your depression. Dealing with cognitive distortions means that you have to be aware of them and then reframe the thoughts associated with them. This all starts with first knowing which distortions you struggle with. Once you know which ones you've experienced, then follow these directions:

1. Make a list and write down the cognitive distortions you think you've experienced.

2. Write down the thoughts you've had for each distortion. Consider adding the events surrounding those thoughts if you remember them.

3. Write down what evidence there is to support or disprove the cognitive distortion.

4. Using the evidence, rewrite your thoughts and create an alternative.

5. Bring awareness to how you feel after examining the original thought, your evidence, and your alternative thoughts. You'll probably feel better once you've realized that your original thought was not based on evidence.

6. Keep on practicing this task. Use a journal to maintain a record, and keep going through it. The goal is to eventually be able to do this inside your own mind by recognizing cognitive distortions as you think them.

Another activity you can try to help you overcome cognitive distortions is to work on understanding the difference between fact and opinion. To do this, make a list of your thoughts and events surrounding them. Take some time to then go through them. Which ones are your opinion (not based on actual evidence) and which ones are fact? Working through this can help you understand how your thoughts are not actually fact and are not always based on reality. Instead, look for the reality of the situation, rather than how your thoughts and beliefs distort the situation. For example, let's say that you're driving down the road and someone cuts you off. You get really angry and then you may take it personally. You may think that they cut you off because you're a slow driver, and they needed to avoid your poor driving skills. If we look at this from a reality/fact perspective, then the facts are this: A person chose to cut you off. That's it. Those are the only facts. The rest is conjecture and opinion. You don't actually know their motivation for cutting you off. Maybe they just drive like that normally, or maybe they're late for work. Whatever their reasoning, you don't know what it is, and you're unlikely to know what it is. So it's important to take the time to observe your situation and separate your thoughts, which are opinions, versus the facts of the situation. This can help you handle cognitive distortions and make corrections.

Both of these repair techniques are ones that will help you regulate your mood after an event. You may choose to continue to feel depressed based on the event, but by challenging your cognitive distortions, you can come to a point where you realize that the event doesn't mean the end of the world and that one negative thing in your life doesn't mean that you're a worthless person.

Relaxation techniques

Relaxation is universal and can really help your sympathetic nervous system calm down by activating your vagus nerve. We've already covered some relaxation techniques in the other chapters, but we'll look at some others here. In general, some things that might help you relax are activities like gardening, mindfulness, or other things that generally feel very relaxing for you. In this case, we're not talking about activities like video games or watching TV. Relaxation techniques are ones that require you to focus on something else beyond entertainment, which can be very passive.

Gardening can be a weird choice for relaxation since it requires work and can be considered exercise. However, it's been used effectively for treating depression and PTSD. This is because gardening requires you to put your focus on a specific activity while also stretching and experiencing different stimuli around you. Being in nature can help calm your heart rate and breathing, also resulting in improved vagus nerve activity. Just being out in sunlight can help ease the symptoms of depression. There are so many reasons why gardening can be very helpful.

One of the reasons why gardening can help is because it engages your social mind. In a way, it requires you to care for something that isn't going to judge you. It's also not a huge caregiving requirement, so there isn't stress associated in that way. Having to care for plants can make you feel like you're being productive. Just caring for a plant can give you a sense of accomplishment. Beyond the social aspects of being a plant caregiver, there is also the fact that many gardens are community-based, resulting in engagement with other people in your community. I have found by and large that gardeners tend to be very kind, supportive people and a lot of us get into gardening to help with our own mental health challenges. You can find a supportive tribe within a garden and that can also help you with your feelings of depression.

When you're gardening by yourself, you won't be engaged with the community so much, but it gives you the perfect opportunity to explore mindfulness in the garden. Using your five senses, you can take the time to focus on the nature around you, resulting in further calm and relaxation. If you want a specific nature meditation script, check out the one in the chapter on trauma. You could use that to help with your depressive symptoms.

If this sounds like something that you're interested in, but you don't have a garden space or don't know what to plant, don't worry. You can create a garden anywhere, including indoors. Some indoor plants that can be great first-time plants are the snake plant, Boston fern, or parlor palm. For outdoor plants, try planting strawberries, lettuce, or most herbs. These can all grow in pots, and they're all fairly easy to grow while requiring you to get your hands dirty. The added benefit of growing herbs or vegetables is that you can literally eat the fruits of your labor, which can be really exciting.

While there are so many benefits to be gained from gardening, it's not for everyone. In that case, try another relaxation technique like mindfulness meditation. Mindfulness meditation can really help with symptoms of depression because it uses breathing and muscle relaxation to create a sense of calm in your body. There are many different kinds of mindfulness you can try, but mindfulness focused on breathing can be very helpful when feeling depressed. There are a couple of different ways you can do to this type of mindfulness. Many people like to simply focus on their inhales and exhales or their natural breathing pattern. To do this style of meditation, here are the steps:

- Find a calm, safe place where you can relax. You can sit or lay down. Simply position yourself in a comfortable way.

- Closing your eyes, place your hands on your stomach and start to focus on your regular breathing pattern. You don't have to change your breathing pattern, just experience it as it is.

- Feel yourself inhale and exhale. Focus on how your body feels with each inhale and exhale.

- Try to maintain your focus on this movement of your breath. As your mind wanders, bring it back to focusing on your breath. You may also notice other body sensations. That's okay. Observe and be aware of your body.

- Keep breathing and maintaining awareness of each breath. If your mind wanders, don't judge, just bring it back to your breathing.

- When you are feeling calm and relaxed, take one deep breath in and let it out through your mouth. Open your eyes and continue with your day.

In this meditation, the focus was purely on our normal body reactions. It wasn't about changing physiology in any way, just being present with our body as is. This can be very calming because it takes us out of our own heads and worries, and instead focuses us on something that we do well, breathing. If you want a meditation that focuses on a specific type of breathing, then here is one that uses number counts to help with breathing focus. This meditation is different from the counted breaths meditation in the chapter on anxiety. That one had long inhales and exhales. This one has a very short inhale and long exhale. The first couple breaths may feel like you're running out of oxygen as you exhale, but keep following through and your body will soon adapt. You can use a metronome to help you remember your counts if you need to. This breathing pattern follows a 2-2-10-2 pattern.

- Find a calm, safe place where you can relax. You can sit or lay down. Simply position yourself in a comfortable way, where you are unlikely to fall asleep.

- Closing your eyes, place your hands on your knees if sitting, or on your stomach if lying down, and start to focus on your breathing.

- When ready take your first inhale, counting to two. Pause for two counts.

- Exhale for 10 counts. Pause for two counts.

- Inhale for two counts. Pause for two counts.

- Exhale for 10 counts. Pause for two counts.

- Continue the pattern for 5-10 minutes.

- Bring awareness to your body and how it feels. Start from your head and continue to your toes. What do you feel physically? Observe them without changing them. If you are feeling discomfort in areas in your body, shift a little to ease the discomfort. Listen to your body for 5 minutes.

- When you're ready to end your meditation, slowly open your eyes and extend your inhale and shorten your exhale.

This mindfulness activity requires you to focus on your breathing and body, but also to change your physiology. By changing your breathing pattern like this, you're activating your vagus nerve, reducing your heart rate, and thus achieving calm. This activity may not work for people who are uncomfortable with body awareness, but it can be adapted to your own personal situations.

If mindfulness meditation is not for you, then find another way to relax and be mindful. Here are some ideas:

- Take a long bath with the purpose of relaxing, not necessarily getting clean. While you are soaking, take some time to categorize your five senses. What are some things that you feel? What do you see and hear? What do you smell and taste? Keep coming back to these things and the feelings of being in the bath. Feel the water around you. Regularly bring your awareness to this moment, not to your emotions, just to your present awareness.

- Go for a walk at sunset. Following the same pattern as above, take some time to categorize your five senses. What animals can you hear? What do you see and smell? What do you feel physically? And what do you taste? Bring your awareness to your current environment and your present moment without focusing on your thoughts. Simply observe.

- Snuggle with a pet that is snuggly. No hedgehogs please, but dogs, cats, and rabbits can make excellent pet choices for snuggling. If you're okay with reptiles, and they're okay with you, then large pet snakes are also great snugglers. Notice the way that your body reacts to snuggling with a pet. Does your breathing deepen? Do your muscles relax? How do you feel emotionally, receiving this unconditional love from an animal? Bring awareness to this feeling.

You can find other activities that bring you relaxation, but remember to choose ones where you're focused on your body sensations, and less on ones that are mindless.

Exercise

Physical activity has always been prescribed by doctors who are treating depression. This is because exercise changes your heart rate and breathing patterns to then help regulate your mood within your brain. When feeling depressed, getting up to exercise can honestly feel like you have to climb a giant mountain. It can be exhausting and unmotivating, and there are honestly some days when you don't want to do anything. Respect those days, but try to move a little. Like walk from one side of your house to the other if possible, or raise your arms above your head and stretch to the side. On days when you're feeling a bit better, try doing some exercise. Doing even a little bit of exercise when feeling depressed can help you feel better. Do as little as you want, and don't feel guilty or judgy about not doing more. Even just five minutes of stretching is great. Some exercise types that are perfect, even if you're not a person who exercises, are yoga, walking, and biking. You don't have to go outside for these activities if you don't want to or if your depression is making it hard for you to socially engage.

Yoga has been linked with easing the symptoms of depression for quite a long time. This is probably because it takes you out of your own head and instead focuses on following a flow. It also requires your breathing to change, which can help with activating your vagus nerve. If you're new to yoga, then start with small stretches and poses. Don't just jump into an advanced pose and hope for the best. There are a lot of yoga videos on YouTube that you can take advantage of. If you're feeling up to it, then going to a yoga class can be a great option, since it will provide you with some social engagement on top of the physical activity. Remember that you don't have to do an hour-long session unless you want to. Spending 5 or 10 minutes doing yoga on days when your depression hits you can be helpful.

Walking is also a good physical activity to try when you're feeling depressed. If you can get the energy up for it, running is even better. If you're struggling with the motivation to do any sort of activity, then try walking around your house in laps. While you walk you can try to categorize the things you see. Just take your mind away from your negative thoughts and focus outward while you walk. If you're feeling more willing, then walk outside. This is a great opportunity because it will provide you with more stimuli while also providing you with sunlight, depending on when you choose to walk. Being exposed to more sunlight can help your mood improve while you focus on your activity. If you can, walk briskly for about 30 minutes. If it's less, that's okay, just try to walk when you can. Running is also a great option because it increases your heart rate more than just walking will. You can walk or run inside your house using a treadmill if you don't feel comfortable being outside or at a gym. Either way, walking and running can give you some relief when you're struggling with depression.

Biking is often a favorite activity because it is often low impact and can feel very freeing. It raises your heart rate and deepens your breathing, just like other exercises, but it also gives you the chance to move at great speeds and distances all on the power of your legs. Biking can be a great way to get outside, and even if you're not doing it for fun, you could bike to work to gain some benefits from it. If you're not really feeling like you want to bike far, then don't. During my own bought of depression, I didn't feel like going to any of the trails I normally bike on. I didn't feel like doing much, in fact, but I dragged myself out to my bike and literally just rode on my driveway. That's all I could manage to bring myself to do, but it helped. Even a little bit of exercise like this can help you improve your mood and your mood regulation. Biking can be done outside or inside if you have a bike trainer stand. Either way, give it a try and see if it's something that you'll like.

If none of these types of physical activity appeal to you, then find something that does. It doesn't have to be anything strenuous unless that's exactly what you want. Gardening counts as physical activity, so if that's what you want to do, then do it. Some people enjoy dancing, which can help with depressed feelings. Others have access to horses and go riding as a way to help. All three of these activities have more benefits than just physical activity. Gardening is naturally very mindful, dancing can be a great way to express your emotions in a creative manner, and horseback riding gives you the opportunity to connect with an animal that is very loving and affectionate. Even walking your dogs can be a great way to get some physical activity in your life. Whatever you chose, involve some movement in your life when you're depressed. Just the smallest bit of activity can do wonders and give you the chance to succeed at something when you're feeling low.

To conclude this chapter, depression is something that affects many adults in the U.S. It can be debilitating and reduce your functioning in your social, work, or school life. However, there are things you can do to help you relieve your depression symptoms. Doing activities that stimulate your vagus nerve and the mood-regulating areas of your brain can help you feel better. Activities like challenging your cognitive distortions, meditation or relaxation, and exercise can all help your symptoms. If you are struggling with a significant amount of depression or are feeling suicidal, then talk to someone. You can always talk anonymously to the National Crisis Call Line if you live in the U.S. Their number is 1-800-273-8255. They can help by giving you support. If you want to work with a therapist or doctor, most are familiar with depression and will also be able to help you manage your symptoms. They may prescribe you medications that can help you regulate your mood, or they may even suggest an implant that directly stimulates your vagus nerve, resulting in a better mood. Whichever path you choose, know that your self-help techniques are always an asset that you can use to help reduce your feelings of depression.

Chapter 6: Stress, Inflammation, and Vagal Tone

In case you haven't realized it by now, many aspects of the mental health discussion above were related to stress. Anxiety causes a stressful response. Trauma reactions are often literally severe stress reactions. And depression causes a different type of stress that makes us want to shut down. All of these reactions result in a more suppressed vagus nerve, which means that we remain in a state of alertness. Our sympathetic nervous system stays active long after it should shut off. Knowing how to activate the vagus nerve can help us reduce our stress responses in so many different kinds of situations. Because stress is involved in inflammation and poor sleep habits, we'll discuss all three in this chapter. We'll also discuss how our body reacts to these situations and how activating the ventral vagus nerve can help us reduce our stress and inflammation while improving our sleep.

Stress

Imagine that you're at work, plugging away and completing what you're supposed to. Suddenly your boss sends you a message requesting that you complete these other items by the end of the day. You can handle it, so you take on those additional tasks. Within the next few minutes, you realize that they're a whole lot larger than you thought they were going to be, so you start to feel overwhelmed. Maybe an hour later, your child's school calls, saying that little Kate is sick and needs to go home. Suddenly you have a full plate with work and a sick child to care for, and your original feeling of being overwhelmed is now a full-blown feeling of being stressed.

Your body starts to release all of these hormones that increase your feelings of stress. Your blood pressure rises, your heart rate increases, and your muscles get tense. This is your sympathetic nervous system coming online to help you deal with the dangerous situation. However, there isn't any actual danger, just a lot of work. Your brain, though, sees this situation as dangerous and puts you in the beginning stages of fight or flight, causing your ventral vagus nerve to retreat. Eventually, once your work is completed and little Kate is better, your brain will tell your ventral vagus that the threat has passed, and your vagus nerve will hit the brakes on your stress response, giving you feelings of calm and well-being, while reducing your heart rate and breathing rate.

This feeling is probably familiar to you. You may not even be aware of the changes in your physiology until you've been stressed for a while. By that point, you've been operating in a high alert state for a bit and then need your vagus nerve to step in. But if your brain still thinks there's a threat, then it won't. The fact is that your body will reactivate its sympathetic nervous system again and again anytime it perceives a threat, including just feeling overwhelmed at work. This frequent activation of being always on alert can do damage to your body. Your heart can start to feel strain, your hormones can cause your blood pressure to remain high, and you are at more risk for cardiovascular issues and obesity. If you experience high amounts of stress every day, then this is how your body responds to it.

Inflammation

Inflammation is when your body decides that it needs to protect itself from attack. This could be from diseases, bacteria, or wounds. You're probably already familiar with experiencing inflammation. If you've ever had a cut on your body, you will have noticed how the area turned red and was painful. This was your body's natural inflammatory response to help heal your body after the wound. It doesn't matter how big or small your wound is, your body tries to heal it through inflammation. You would have also experienced inflammation whenever you've been sick with the flu or similar disease. Your body responds to diseases by increasing your body temperature, flaring up pain signals, and sending white blood cells to combat whatever is causing the issue. While all of this is to your benefit since it can help with healing, too much inflammation can also be very negative.

Having too much of an inflammatory response means that your body starts to focus on areas that either don't need healing or do, but the inflammation causes the problems to worsen. This results in chronic, debilitating pain. Rheumatoid arthritis is one example of a severe inflammatory response that does more damage than good. Perhaps, unsurprisingly, having negative inflammatory responses can be triggered by stress.

Inflammation and stress go together hand-in-hand. Chronic stress can trigger your body to start an inflammatory response. When you're feeling stressed all the time, your body gets used to the hormones released and 'numb' to the ones released to help you heal. Because your body gets used to its stress hormones, it becomes less responsive to the inflammatory ones that are trying to heal it. This can lead to your body being more impacted by diseases. If your inflammatory response isn't working well because of stress, this means that you're more susceptible to colds, fevers, and diseases.

Because stress and inflammation are related, that means that you can work on them both by activating your vagus nerve. So if you reduce your stress by activating your vagus nerve, you'll also be able to reduce your inflammation. Surprisingly, scientists have found that implants that trigger stimulation of the vagus nerve do help with reduced inflammation, particularly with inflammation like arthritis. Stress and inflammation are both connected to your vagus nerve and vagal tone.

Vagal Tone

Vagal tone is how your vagus nerve is measured based on its connection with your heart rate. It is an indication of how well your vagus nerve is working. Your vagus nerve regulates your heart rate by slowing it down during your exhales. So as you inhale, your heart speeds up, and as you exhale, your heart slows down. This improves your vagal tone and reduces your blood pressure, makes you feel calm, and keeps you in that 'rest and digest stage.' Needless to say, anything that affects your heart will then affect your vagus nerve. And stress is a well-known disease that affects your heart.

Stress lowers your vagal tone or reduces the activation of your vagus nerve. Because this shifts your vagus nerve, it means that it also changes how your heart rate changes. This leads to you having a faster heart rate and an increase in physical illness. A lower vagal tone is associated with all of the mental struggles we discussed earlier, and it's also attached to cardiovascular disease, stroke, and more. So having a lower vagal tone is not the best for your body. Conversely, having a higher vagal tone results in you having better well-being.

Now you may be wondering why vagal tone is discussed here at this point of the book. The reason is this: By this point in the book, you should be able to see how everything is interconnected. Stress changes your vagal tone which changes your emotional regulation. Emotional regulation is part of the struggle of dealing with depression. Trauma creates a massive stress response to the environment, which lowers your vagal tone and results in your vagus nerve going into 'freeze' more often than it should, while also increasing your sympathetic nervous response. Anxiety is the same, as it causes stress which reduces your vagal tone, which in turn causes more anxiety. It's all interconnected in a cycle that keeps being perpetuated between your environment, brain, and vagus nerve. The only way to break the cycle is to activate your vagus nerve and improve your vagal tone. Every self-help technique discussed so far does this. In the next chapter, we are going to look at additional techniques that can help reduce your stress response and improve your vagal tone.

Chapter 7: Techniques to Activate Your Vagus Nerve

Within each of the chapters discussing mental well-being, there have been a variety of self-help techniques discussed. Each of these techniques helps with activating your vagus nerve and improving your vagal tone. Each of them also works to reduce your state of alertness and help you reach a state of equilibrium, while also working on your mental well-being. In this chapter, we will look at additional techniques that can be used anytime you need to activate your vagus nerve. Some of them can work for anxiety, trauma, and depression, but some won't. If you want to focus on activating your vagus nerve for those issues, then use the self-help suggested in those chapters first before exploring with these ones. Some of these techniques may make trauma symptoms worse, so proceed with caution. These techniques are excellent for reducing some of your generalized stress and activating your vagus nerve to feel better. Try a few out and make a list of 'go-to' strategies that you can rely on in the event that you feel overwhelmed by your sympathetic nervous system.

Breathing Techniques

Throughout this book, we've talked about breathing techniques. This is because breathing is intimately related to your heart rate and vagal tone. Deep, long breaths reduce your heart rate and improve your vagal tone, so it makes sense that breathing patterns can be used to activate your parasympathetic nervous system. This, in turn, creates a feeling of calmness and safety, while also improving your decision-making skills. There are three breathing techniques that you can try to improve your vagal tone. They are diaphragmatic breathing, alternate nose breathing, and what is fondly known as Darth Vader breathing, or the Ujjayi breath.

Diaphragmatic breathing requires you to fully expand and contract your diaphragm. Your diaphragm is the band of muscles beneath your lungs. Its spasms are what cause hiccups, and when you use it for breathing, you'll feel your stomach expand, rather than your chest or shoulders. When you first start this exercise, try it while lying down, as it might feel easier for you. As you get used to it, you can try doing it while sitting up in a chair.

- Lie down in a comfortable position. It's a good idea to place a pillow behind your knees for added comfort.

- Place one hand on your stomach so you can feel its movements, and the other hand on your chest.

- As you inhale, breathe deeply, expanding your stomach. You should feel your belly rise with your hands.

- As you exhale, purse your lips (as if you were going to whistle) and release your exhale through your mouth. Use your diaphragm to expel the air. Your belly should decrease as you breathe out.

- Throughout this process, you should feel the hand on your chest stay mostly still and the hand on your belly move up and down.

- Repeat this process 5-10 times as you need it. You'll get better at it as you keep practicing the technique.

In this kind of breathing, your pursed lips help to control how much you're exhaling. So your exhale will be long and slow, something that will help to activate your vagus nerve. You should try to do diaphragmatic breathing several times a day. Since it's a short exercise, it won't take up too much of your time. For a longer exercise, consider one of the other breathing techniques below.

Alternate nostril breathing is another technique that can help you feel calm. While it doesn't include long exhales, it does restrict some of your air movement, which can be very calming.

It can also help you be mindful as you breathe, and mindfulness is another activity that can improve vagal tone. Alternate nostril breathing means inhaling through one nostril and exhaling out of the other nostril. You use your fingers to block the nostril you're not using. So, for example, if you are inhaling through your right nostril, then you'll block the left. Then as you exhale, release the left nostril and block the right so all of your air comes out of only one nostril. You'll move back and forth between the two. You only want to do this for about 5-30 minutes in your day, and you can vary how long you're inhaling and exhaling while practicing this. The point is to remain mindful as you breathe, following your pattern of one nostril to inhale, and one to exhale.

- Sit in a comfortable position with your back straight and your hands resting gently on your lap.

- Shape your right hand into the 'hand loose' or shaka position, where your thumb and pinky are out, and your other three fingers are curled into your palm.

- Raise your right hand to your face before your nose. You will use your thumb and pinky to close your nostrils.

- Completely exhale before using your thumb to close your right nostril.

- Inhale through your left nostril and then close your left nostril with your pinky.

- Release your thumb and exhale through your right nostril.

- Inhale through your right nostril. Close your right nostril with your thumb.

- Release your pinky and exhale through your left nostril.

- Keep following the pattern, exhaling and inhaling out of one nostril before switching to the next.

While you may look a little strange when doing alternate nostril breathing, ignore the strange glances and focus on its many key benefits. Not only does it change your breathing pattern but it reduces your stress levels and improves your cardiovascular health. This, in turn, improves your vagal tone. It lowers your heart rate, breathing rate, and your blood pressure. All of these are crucial benefits to improving your well-being.

Ujjayi breathing is the last technique we'll cover in this section. This style of breathing requires you to focus on your body, specifically your throat, and focus on the sound you make. It's often called Darth Vader breathing because if you're doing it right, you'll probably sound like Darth Vader as you exhale. Or if you want a more peaceful analogy, you'll sound like the ocean as you exhale. The Ujjayi breath causes a long, deep exhale that helps you feel relaxed and also activates your vagus nerve. If you practice yoga, then you can use the Ujjayi breath during your practice. You can also use it when sitting or relaxing as well.

- Sit in a comfortable position with your back straight and your hands laying gently in your lap.

- Relax your jaw and mouth, letting your mouth open a little. Your inhales will come in through your nose and go out through your mouth.

- Inhale and exhale gently, paying attention to the movement of the air from your nose to your windpipe to your lungs and back up to your mouth.

- On your next exhale, sigh. Make the noise you do when you sigh, or act like you are trying to fog up a window.

- Pay attention to how your palate and throat change as you exhale. They should have a slight constriction.

- Keep inhaling and exhaling, sighing with every exhale, getting familiar with that feeling of constriction.

- When you feel comfortable and familiar with the sensation in your throat, try closing your mouth and now exhaling from your nose, maintaining the same feeling in your throat. You should be making a sound like the ocean or like Darth Vader.

- Continue your practice for 5-15 minutes.

- Each breath should be smooth and slow. If you feel like your throat is tight, finish your practice and breath normally.

The Ujjayi breath is a great way to feel calm, but it can cause you to feel discomfort. If this happens, then release the breath and follow your normal breathing pattern. In fact, for all of these breathing patterns, if you feel discomfort, lightheadedness, or faintness, then stop the practice and return to your normal breathing pattern. If none of these breathing patterns work for you, that's okay. There is a myriad of other ways that you can relax.

Mindfulness Meditation

We've already discussed some of the great benefits of mindfulness meditation. It can help you focus on your present moment and make you more aware of your body. It can bring awareness to physical sensations you would have ignored before. All of this can help you further understand your physical reactions to stress and know ways of bringing relaxation to your body. There are many different ways you can approach meditation. Choose the one that you're the most comfortable with.

One mindfulness meditation that can really help with stress, anxiety, and depression is loving-kindness mindfulness. This is because it creates more positive emotions which, in turn, change your body physiology and help you improve your vagal tone. In fact, loving-kindness can help you overcome any issues with low mood or low self-esteem. They can also help you with emotions like anger, guilt, and resentment. All of these involve our feelings about ourselves or others. Loving-kindness is about reminding yourself of kindness to you and to others. It creates so many positive emotions that it can change your mentality going forward and is a great way to start changing your cognitive distortions.

To start your loving-kindness meditation, you're going to need a safe, comfortable space. Since this meditation is kind of long, you may want to have this book open while you do it, or you can listen to a guided meditation to walk you through it. This loving-kindness meditation is based on the work of Dr. Emma Seppala.

1. Start by sitting cross-legged if you can or sitting on a chair. Relax your body, and close your eyes so that you are focused on your internal world, rather than the external one.

2. Take a deep breath in and slowly release it.

3. Think about someone who is close to you and loves you. This can be someone from your life now, someone from the past, or someone who has passed away. Imagine that person standing beside you. They are sending you their love and their hopes for your happiness and safety. See and feel the warm wishes coming from that person toward you. You might picture it as a wave coming toward you, filling you, and surrounding you.

4. Think about a second person who also loves you. They also send you their love and their hopes for your happiness and safety. See and feel that warmth surround you and enter inside of you.

5. Now, imagine that you are surrounded by all the people you have ever known who love and cherish you. Your friends, family members, and community. They are sending you their love and their hopes for your happiness and safety. Surround yourself in that love and fill your heart and body with it. You are overfilled with love.

6. Look at the first person next to you. Start to send them your love. You and this person are alike; you both wish for happiness and love. Send your love and your hopes for their happiness and safety to them.

7. Silently repeat this phrase three times, sending the wishes to that person.

    a. May you be safe, may you be happy, and may you be healthy.

8. Now focus on the second person on your other side. Start to send them your love. You and this person are alike; you both wish for happiness and love. Send your love and your hopes for their happiness and safety to them.

9. Silently repeat this phrase three times, sending the wishes to that person.

    a. Just like I hope to, may you live a good life full of safety, happiness, and good health.

10. Now imagine all of the other people who love you. Start to send them your love. You are all alike; you all wish for happiness and love. Send your love and your hopes for their happiness to them.

11. Silently repeat this phrase three times, sending wishes to those people.

    a. May your life be full of happiness, well-being, and health.

12. Think of an acquaintance that you know. Someone that you have no particular feelings toward. You are all alike; you both wish for happiness and well-being. Send all of your hopes for their well-being to them.

13. Silently repeat this phrase three times, sending the wishes to that person.

    a. Just like I hope to, may you live a good life with health and happiness.

14. Think of another acquaintance who you know, but don't have any particular feelings toward. You are all alike; you both wish for happiness and well-being. Send all of your hopes for their well-being to them.

15. Silently repeat this phrase three times, sending the wishes to that person.

    a. May your life be full of happiness and well-being.

16. Now imagine the whole world in front of you. All of the living beings in the world are just like you; they all want to be happy. Send all of your warm wishes to them.

17. Silently repeat this phrase three times, sending your wishes to every living being in the world.

    a. May your life be full of happiness and well-being.

18. Gently bring your awareness back to yourself. Take a deep breath in and then out. Bring awareness to your body and mind. Think about how you feel after doing this meditation. Open your eyes and continue your day.

Once you've completed the meditation, you should feel a little better. You may feel relaxed and calm. You may even feel more compassion for others. If you don't, that's okay. Keep practicing loving-kindness meditation to gain the benefits from it. If this isn't your cup of tea, try some other kinds of meditation. If you want a more physical kind of meditation, try yoga, qigong, or taiji (thai chi).

Yoga is often considered to be very relaxing as it uses movements and breathing to help calm the body. It can sometimes be triggering for people, so if you've experienced trauma or PTSD, proceed with caution or do yoga with someone who understands trauma. There is some evidence that yoga can stimulate the parasympathetic nervous system and the vagus nerve. It's also been linked with helping to heal depression, anxiety, stress, and chronic pain. So it can be worth it to try if you want to activate your vagus nerve.

There are a lot of different types of yoga to try. If you've been practicing yoga for a while, then stick with the ones you know or try something new. If you're a beginner, then don't start with the advanced classes. Here are some great types of yoga that are good for beginners but also help with stress reduction.

Hatha Yoga - In a hatha yoga class, you'll can a basic understanding of the different poses in yoga. It's generally considered to be a gentle yoga class and shouldn't strain you too much. You'll learn to work on posture, while also following the breath.

Iyengar Yoga- This type of yoga is very focused on your posture and poses. There isn't a lot of strenuous work, but you'll have to maintain poses for a while. The classes should be run by someone who understands the human body well and can provide you with support in different positions. If you choose to do Iyengar yoga, make sure that your instructor has been well-trained and can provide you with the necessary guidance so you don't hurt yourself.

Restorative Yoga - Like the name itself suggests, restorative yoga is all about relaxation. In this style of yoga, you put yourself in poses while being supported by other materials. So while you are in the pose, you're not actually straining yourself

Each of these kinds of yoga can require a class with an instructor. However, if you don't want to go to an actual class, then you can find some good yoga videos online. For rest and relaxation, choose yoga videos that use terms like gentle yoga, beginner's yoga, or yoga for relaxation. Find videos that you enjoy and help you relax. If gentle yoga is not your thing, they try vinyasa yoga, ashtanga yoga, or Bikram yoga. All of these are more intense, but also put a lot of emphasis on the breath and movement. All of them can help you achieve more balance in your body.

Qigong is a very interesting type of meditation. It combines physical form and movement with focused breathing and meditation. Its goal is to balance your life energy, or Qi. It has a lot of backing from both traditional medicine and modern science. Many scientists consider qigong to promote well-being. It causes relaxation of your muscles, reduces your stress levels, and deepens your breathing, which, as has been repeated many times thus far, can help with activating your vagus nerve. Qigong has many different forms, and because of this, it can be adapted for many different people. It's often used medically in China, is related to many different types of martial arts, and is sometimes just simple meditation and movement. One of the most well-known forms of qigong in the U.S. is tai chi.

If you've ever walked through a park in a major city during the weekday morning, you may come across a group of people doing slow, fluid movements that look very much like martial arts. They're most likely doing tai chi. It is, in fact, a type of martial arts that focuses on the slow movement of the body and breath. It is considered a style of meditation, even though there is an exercise component to it. If you're interested in either qigong or tai chi, find a class near you and give it a try. You can also find videos on YouTube for home practice. Tai chi takes a lot of practice before the flow of it becomes normal, so keep working with it.

Massage

Many people know that massages can help them relax. There's just something so soothing about putting pressure on a point in your body that's painful or tight. There's some research that supports that massages create a physiological response that reduces stress, blood pressure, and heart rate. This then results in an increase in vagal tone. In fact, the vagus remains activated even after a massage has ended. To gain the benefit of a massage, it has to be a moderate pressure massage, not a light massage. This means that you can get a decent massage from a masseuse and gain the benefit of an activated vagus nerve, as well as feeling like you're relaxed enough to sleep on the table. You could also get a massage from a chiropractor, who is there to help you heal. A chiropractor knows exactly how much pressure to apply to your neck, shoulders, and back to gain you the most benefit from the massage. It can be a little painful at first, but the results are always worth it.

If you don't want to see a masseuse or chiropractor, consider giving yourself a massage at home. To get some good pressure, you'll need to use your body weight to help aid the massage. You can use a foam roller that you can lay on to help give yourself a back massage.

- Take the roller, place it on the floor, and lie down on top of the roller with it positioned at your shoulders.

- Using your feet to propel you, roll back and forth on the roller.

- Your body weight will push your back into the roller, giving you a significant amount of pressure.

- You can also use it on your lower back, thighs, legs, chest, etc.

A foam roller or massage roller are great options for giving yourself a massage at home. If you don't have a foam roller, that's okay. Try using a tennis ball if you have one. A tennis ball will give you some resistance, while also give you a strong pressure point. If you want to massage your shoulders, place the tennis ball against your shoulder and then lean back against a wall. The tennis ball should be between your shoulder and the wall. Then move your body like Baloo from *The Jungle Book* does; move up and down, using your knees and legs to shift you. You can also move side to side as necessary. The tennis ball will give you a lot of pressure, so be prepared for that and keep going until you feel your muscles relax. Then move to the next shoulder. When using a tennis ball, it's important that you don't put it over your spine. This can cause you significant pain. Make sure that it's just on your shoulders on either side of your spine.

You can also use a tennis ball on your feet, hands, thighs, or legs. Just use your body weight to apply a good amount of pressure.

Reflexology is another type of massage that can reduce your stress and increased vagal activity. It's actually something that's been around for millennia and can be considered as part of traditional medicine. In reflexology, the feet are connected to parts of the body and putting pressure on them results in healing to that part of the body. In general, reflexology is done with the feet, but it can also be done to the hands or ears. You can go to a specialist if you want to, but if you want to approach reflexology yourself and do it for yourself, then you can. You'll simply need to have some lotion or body oil that you like, and a reflexology chart that can be found online.

- Using the chart, you're going to take your thumb and apply pressure to the area of your foot, hand, or ear which corresponds to the chosen organ on the chart.

- Apply pressure and move your thumb in a circular motion before shifting it slightly into a new position.

- Make sure you cover the entire area that you need for that organ.

- If the area is large, go over it a couple of times, moving back and forth across the area on your foot or hand. If the area is small, just spend some time focusing on that area.

- The pressure you apply should be as strong as you can while remaining comfortable. You want there to be a moderate amount of pressure.

Working with a reflexologist can give you even more benefits since they have received the training necessary to pinpoint areas that you want to be stimulated. They also know exactly how much pressure needs to be applied to those areas. That being said, you can always do some reflexology at home for your added benefit.

Acupuncture

Acupuncture is an ancient way of healing your body. It involves a lot of needles, though they don't go deep and don't cause too much pain. Acupuncture can help you with stress reduction and mood improvement. But the best part is how acupuncture on your ear can stimulate your vagus nerve. It can help you calm your mind from anxiety, reduce your heart rate and maintain your rate pattern, and help with your mental health. While it sounds really terrifying, it's actually not that scary. Ear acupuncture, called auricular acupuncture, is one on the outside shell of your ear. It doesn't go inside your ear canal at all, so there is no risk of something sharp and pointy entering your ear.

Each needle is carefully placed to help stimulate specific points that are aligned with your body. That being said, ear acupuncture is not something that you can do on your own. Acupuncture, in general, should be given by someone who has received a lot of training and also maintains the hygiene of their workspace.

Change Your Diet

Changing your diet can give you many physical benefits, but it can also help you activate your vagus nerve. In general, you want to eat heart-healthy foods since your heart is connected to the vagus nerve. Heart-healthy foods include whole grains, fruits, vegetables, and oily fish. Some of these foods are rich in omega 3s. Omega 3s can help with your heart rate and vagal tone, so foods rich in it can be very beneficial for your body and vagus nerve.

Beyond heart-healthy foods, you should consider adding foods that help your gut microbiota. This hasn't been touched on in a while, but remember how your vagus nerve is connected to your gut so that you have a visceral response to your environment? Well, improving your gut microbiota can help with increasing your vagus response. Foods with probiotics in them can be especially helpful. Probiotics were found to help people regulate their mood and reduce their stress and cortisol levels (Breit et al., 2018). So consider adding probiotic foods like yogurt, miso, and kimchi to your diet. All of these can help you improve your vagal tone and reduce your stress levels.

Supportive Relationships

The final self-help technique for improving your vagal tone is to create and maintain supportive relationships. This is because there is an interconnection between the vagus and our social responses. When the polyvagal theory was discussed earlier, it was mentioned how the ventral vagus was our means for social engagement. Because of this, if we want to improve our vagal tone, then making social connections can help. When we have supportive people around us, our ventral vagus nerve remains active and promotes feelings of well-being and safety. So social connections can improve our vagus nerve's response.

Not only can social engagement promote feelings of safety, but it can also give us more positive emotions. Having positive emotions can help with improving vagal tone and vice versa. Because positive emotions are your goal, make sure that you have friends who are genuinely your friends. They should be supportive and loving to you (and vice versa, of course) for everyone to get the most benefit from the relationship. Vagal activation is much stronger in supportive friendships, which means that acquaintances aren't going to give you the same benefits as having close friendships. The stronger the relationship, the better your vagal tone when you're with them. So engaging in strong social relationships is a great way for you to improve your vagus response.

Conclusion

You've reached the end of this book! You've gained the ability to control and activate your vagus nerve to reach a state of calm. The vagus nerve is like a little magic button in your body that you can press anytime you're feeling overwhelmed, stressed, anxious, or depressed. It's one of the key parts of your parasympathetic nervous system and helps to ensure that your sympathetic nervous system doesn't stay active all the time. Activating the vagus nerve isn't hard, and it can be easily done to help you feel calm and safe. Using the techniques mentioned in this book, you can achieve peace and relaxation. You've probably started reading this book to improve your emotions and well-being, and I hope this book has helped you achieve this goal.

References

9 Fascinating Facts About the Vagus Nerve (2018, November 13). Retrieved from http://mentalfloss.com/article/65710/9-nervy-facts-about-vagus-nerve

A., V. der K. B. (2015). The body keeps the score: brain, mind, and body in the healing of trauma. NY, NY: Penguin Books.

American Psychiatric Association (2013). Diagnostic and statistical manual of mental disorders (5th ed.). Arlington: American Psychiatric Publishing.

Auricular Acupuncture (n.d.). Retrieved from https://www.sciencedirect.com/topics/medicine-and-dentistry/auricular-acupuncture

Bergland, C. (2014). How Does the Vagus Nerve Convey Gut Instincts to the Brain? Retrieved from https://www.psychologytoday.com/us/blog/the-athletes-way/201405/how-does-the-vagus-nerve-convey-gut-instincts-the-brain

Bergland, C. (2016). Vagus Nerve Stimulation Dramatically Reduces Inflammation. Retrieved from https://www.psychologytoday.com/us/blog/the-athletes-way/201607/vagus-nerve-stimulation-dramatically-reduces-inflammation

Bouguyon, C. (n.d.). What is Qigong? Retrieved from https://www.nqa.org/what-is-qigong-

Breit, S., Kupferberg, A., Rogler, G., & Hasler, G. (2018). Vagus Nerve as Modulator of the Brain–Gut Axis in Psychiatric and Inflammatory Disorders. Frontiers in Psychiatry, 9. doi: 10.3389/fpsyt.2018.00044

Cronkleton, E. (2018). Alternate Nostril Breathing. Retrieved from https://www.healthline.com/health/alternate-nostril-breathing

Deans, E. (2013). Depression and a Broken Heart. Retrieved from https://www.psychologytoday.com/us/blog/evolutionary-psychiatry/201310/depression-and-broken-heart

Field, T. (2006). Massage therapy research methods. Massage Therapy Research, 1–22. doi: 10.1016/b978-0-443-10201-1.50005-2

Gaiam (n.d.). A Beginner's Guide to 8 Major Styles of Yoga. Retrieved from https://www.gaiam.com/blogs/discover/a-beginners-guide-to-8-major-styles-of-yoga

Kok, B. E., Coffey, K. A., Cohn, M. A., Catalino, L. I., Vacharkulksemsuk, T., Algoe, S. B., ... Fredrickson, B. L. (2013).

How Positive Emotions Build Physical Health. Psychological Science, 24(7), 1123–1132. doi: 10.1177/0956797612470827

Loving-Kindness Meditation (Greater Good in Action). (n.d.). Retrieved from https://ggia.berkeley.edu/practice/loving_kindness_meditation

Maddux, J. E., & Winstead, B. A. (2017). Psychopathology. Taylor & Francis.

National Council for Community Behavioral Healthcare (n.d.). How to Manage Trauma. Retrieved from https://www.integration.samhsa.gov/clinical-practice/Trauma-infographic.pdf

Porges, S. W. (2007). The polyvagal perspective. Biological Psychology, 74(2), 116–143. doi: 10.1016/j.biopsycho.2006.06.009

Richardson, M. W. (2019). Are commercial vagus nerve stimulation devices safe and effective? Retrieved from https://www.brainfacts.org/diseases-and-disorders/therapies/2019/are-commercial-vagus-nerve-stimulation-devices-safe-and-effective-042419

Rothschild, B. (2017). The body remembers (Vol. 2). New York: Norton.

Seladi-Schulman, J. (2018, August 27). Vagus Nerve: Anatomy and Function, Diagram, Stimulation, Conditions. Retrieved from https://www.healthline.com/human-body-maps/vagus-nerve

Seymour, T. (n.d.). Vagus nerve: Function, stimulation, and further research. Retrieved from https://www.medicalnewstoday.com/articles/318128.php

Streeter, C., Gerberg, P., Saper, R., Ciraulo, D., & Brown, R. (2012). Effects of yoga on the autonomic nervous system, gamma-aminobutyric-acid, and allostasis in epilepsy, depression, and post-traumatic stress disorder. Medical Hypotheses, 78(5), 571–579. doi: 10.1016/j.mehy.2012.01.021

Tran, P. (2013, September 17). How to Practice Ujjayi Breath in Yoga. Retrieved from https://www.yogaoutlet.com/blogs/guides/how-to-practice-ujjayi-breath-in-yoga

Vagus Nerve (n.d.). Retrieved from https://www.psychologytoday.com/us/basics/vagus-nerve

Wagner, D. (2016, July 9). Polyvagal theory in practice. Retrieved from https://ct.counseling.org/2016/06/polyvagal-theory-practice/#

Wang, Y., Zhao, X., O'Neil, A., Turner, A., Liu, X., & Berk, M. (2013). Altered cardiac autonomic nervous function in depression. BMC Psychiatry, 13(1). doi: 10.1186/1471-244x-13-187

What is the vagus nerve? (2017, October 23). Retrieved from https://www.okheart.com/about-us/ohh-news/what-is-the-vagus-nerve

Made in the USA
Middletown, DE
08 January 2020